Master Samuel Scott
The Bully Problem

Master Samuel Scott
The Bully Problem

THE BULLY PROBLEM

DON'T LEAVE YOUR CHILD'S FUTURE IN THE HANDS OF A BULLY

LIST OF BOOKS WRITTEN BY THE AUTHOR

Women's Personal Safety 101 (2008)

Life Skills Lessons (2012)

Life Skills Lessons for Teens (2012)

My Journey to Blackbelt (2018)

THE BULLY PROBLEM

DON'T LEAVE YOUR CHILD'S FUTURE IN THE HANDS OF A BULLY

MASTER SAMUEL SCOTT

Master Samuel Scott
The Bully Problem

Testimonials

For more than 30 years Samuel Scott's life has been marked by his deep well of human compassion and knowledge. This deep well of knowledge and compassion has been honed and applied through real life teaching and training sessions and it's about time that the whole world gets in on this proven process that can stop bullying everywhere. **(Darrell Green, Pro Football Hall of Fame, Associate Athletic Director George Mason University)**

I have had the pleasure of working with Samuel Scott over the years as he has helped countless men, women, and children empower themselves in the art of self defense. Unfortunately, we live in a time when it is absolutely vital to know how to protect ourselves against would-be assailants who rob us of our sense of safety. I am so delighted to know that Samuel is taking his skills now a step further to address the growing problem of bullying. "The Bully Problem" is the tool every parent must have in their arsenal before they send their children off to school.
(Renee J. Nash, Director of News and Public Affairs WHUR 96.3FM & SiriusXM 141 HUR Voices)

This book is absolutely paramount to the lives of parents and children everywhere. Its timing is impeccable as currently more than 1 out of every 5 students report being bullied while at school, many having this pattern continue beyond the campus. This book takes head-on the stark reality of bullying and its traumatizing effect on our children. It then challenges us to become part of the solution to this overreaching problem. Thank you Master Samuel Scott for your selfless leadership, tireless commitment and masterful training. With the addition of this book, you have facilitated an unparalleled opportunity for children to not only survive but actually overcome the lingering effects of bullying. I highly recommend this book.
(Gwendolyn R. Manning, Black Infant Health, Program Director, Long Beach, CA)

Grandmaster Scott is tackling this issue of bullying head on and from every angle. Master Scott is not only discussing a crucial issue that greatly effects youth around the country, not only bringing to light and making parents aware of what happens far too often in middle and high schools around the country, but with this book Master Scott will equip youth to be the ambassadors to fight against it. **(Etan Thomas, Author of "We Matter: Athletes and Activism," entrepreneur, and former NBA Wizards player)**

"The Bullying Problem" demonstrates Master Samuel Scott's compassion for today's youth and his commitment to offering viable solutions and strategies that can help eradicate bullying in every community across America. **(Dana Brown, MA, LPC Community Resource Advocate, Prince Georges County, Maryland)**

Master Samuel Scott is a renowned teacher, leader and lectured who is passionate about helping our communities to stay safe and be informed. He has committed his life long work to helping others. I am excited about his new book "The Bully Problem." This book is life changing and it will set your Soul on Fire to educate our schools and communities on this important issue. In fact, every house hold need this book to understand the effects of bullying and how we can change the course of a life. I know that your life will never be the same and will forever be blessed. I count it an honor and privilege to give an acknowledgment of this powerful book from an extraordinary leader. **(Dr. Jacqueline Mohair, Founder of Trinity Girls Network Corp. & Trinity International University of Ambassadors)**

It cannot be overstated the attention that must be focused on the maliciousness of "bullying". It is particularly important that we continue to elevate the discussion of bullying in our homes, schools, churches and the halls of all levels government. It is gratifying that Samuel Scott with his immeasurable tactical and entrepreneurial expertise has written the "Bullying Problem" for people to learn more about this topic. Moreover, he has provided strategies that can be useful for parents, teachers and concerned individuals. **Dr. Justine Bell, Retired Professor Public Administration, California State Dominguez Hills**

Bullying is a serious issue inside and outside of schools in America. This hurtful behavior can have a negative impact on those who are bullied, those who bully, students, parents, families, schools, teachers, administrators, and countless others. Bullying affects others in a multitude of ways. This phenomenon often reveals itself in negative physical and mental issues such as depression, anxiety, loneliness, sadness, sleep/eating disorders and other health complaints causing a marked decrease in academic achievement.

Samuel Scott's book, The Bully Problem, is a common sense guide to identifying, understanding and ultimately banishing the occurrence of bullying. This book will offer the reader effective strategies and techniques to assist on the pathway to survival of the exceptionally prevalent and socially unacceptable practice of bullying others! **(Dr. Janice P. Hay, Retired Principal, Prince George's County MD Public School System)**

Master Samuel Scott is a man of impeccable character and drive. He has put together a well researched book on a topic, (bullying), which continues to hold our future generations of leaders captive. This is a must read book. ***(Robert "Bruce" Ewing, Major (Retired) US Armed Forces, CEO/Founder of Habu Ewing Martial Arts and Fitness Academy)***

To My Mother:

I would like to dedicate this book to my loving mother, the late Thelma Mae Scott, who I call my Master Teacher.

Thank you for giving me a strong foundation from which to grow in the spirit of love and compassion for all. I will share your words of encouragement, compassion, and love for one another to all who will listen.

Lastly, I will continue to be an instrument for The Creator to use as a means to help bring about positive change in this world.

Samuel

Acknowledgments

Photos – Brian Williams

Book Cover Design – Ace Graphics

Assistant Editors – Valencia D. Robinson and
Tonya Alston

TABLE OF CONTENTS

Why This Book (From the Author)

Growing up as a child in a tough neighborhood in Long Island, NY, I not only saw my share of bullying, I was also a victim of bullying. However, the bullying that I experienced and witnessed hardly compares to what children are going through today.

In my day, if a neighbor or stranger observed a child being bullied, they not only intervened but they went to your house and told your parents. Try doing that today, and you might find yourself getting a beat down by the bystanders, friends, or the bully's parents. Instead of helping the victim, kids and adults are edging on these vicious acts of violence. Some even videotape it for the world to see on social media. The concept of "it takes a village to raise a child" is, indeed, a thing of the past. People are either afraid to intervene, hardened by all the violence in society, or simply don't care about one another's safety or wellbeing.

Our homes, which were once considered a haven for our children to escape the vicious abuse of bullying, are now being infiltrated by a new tactic called *cyberbullying*. This cruel approach to bullying has caused a serious surge in teen suicide also known as *bullycide*.

Statistics show that one in five kids are being bullied or are bullies. Meaning, between the neighborhood bullies, school bullies, and now cyberbullying, our children have an even higher chance of being a victim of bullying. Many feel like they have nowhere to turn. With schools being overwhelmed with this growing problem, teachers not being adequately trained to handle this growing epidemic, and parents too busy trying to provide a decent living for their family, our kids are literally being left to fend for themselves.

In January 2017, *USA Today* reported that an 8-year old, named Gabriel Taye, killed himself two days after peers knocked him unconscious in a restroom at Cincinnati's Carson Elementary. The security camera showed other students touched and kicked Gabriel during the incident. For reasons like this, I have spent the last 25 years on the front lines, addressing the bully problem. I know how bullying can drastically affect a child through adulthood.

As a former Correctional Officer, I saw first-hand where many bullies and some victims end up. I clearly remember the day that I first reported for duty as a Correctional Officer. I had pictured in my mind that I would be working with the worst of the worse in society. The men and women who simply decided to take the dark path with no regard for the law, order, or human life. What I wasn't prepared for were the thousands of young boys and girls who had gotten themselves caught up in the legal system. I remember sitting with a group of young inmates and just having a man-to-young-man talk with them. Now, before this meeting, I observed them while they were visiting with their parents and other family members. Most of them had loving parents and family members, so it didn't appear as if their veering off track started at home.

During our meeting, I asked them, "What happened? What made you all decide to pursue a life of crime?" Although there were a few that said, "Nobody really cared about me anyway," most of the responses were, "I was following the 'cool' crowd in our neighborhood and school. They were the popular tough guys that everyone feared and respected. And to keep from getting beat up or bullied, I joined them." Most of them said 'that their parents had no idea what they were doing in the streets.' When I asked them, "How did your parents not know that you were going down this vicious path?" Many stated that their parents were too busy working two jobs, going to school, hanging out, or raising their younger siblings.

As I drilled deeper to get to the root of their feelings and emotions, many began to cry and said that 'they didn't want to hurt anyone, use or sell drugs, but they felt like they had to do it to survive.' They said to me that, "People think it's easy in the streets. All that 'just walk away stuff' doesn't work out here in the real world. You either fight your way out, be their victim or join them. And it's too many to fight your way out, so your only real options are to be a victim or join the crew, period."

Knowing that my own childhood experiences validated their reality, I spent 15 years in the prison system educating and inspiring our young future leaders to commit to transforming their lives. I met with them weekly and brought them books and self-help videos to help inspire and encourage them to change. I am happy to say that many of them made it out of prison and have gone on to become very productive citizens in society.

Although it was my plan since childhood to open my own martial arts school, I truly feel that The Most High placed me in the Correctional System to see with my own eyes the work that was ahead of me. He wanted me to see the true depth of the social issues that affected our young people's future. I also believe that he wanted me to see the gift that He so graciously deposited in me to help inspire and transform lives. That chapter of my life at the Dept. of Corrections solidified my purpose in life.

After 15 years of dedicated service and much prayer, I walked into work one day and resigned, effective immediately. I decided that adding value to our future leaders' lives was my true purpose. This is what gave birth to the opening of my life-skills, character-building martial arts school, Full Circle Martial Arts Academy.

As you read this book, think about your own childhood and how you felt when you (or a friend) were bullied, then multiply it times a hundred! As a student of martial excellence, it is my duty and responsibility to do whatever it takes to help bring an end to this vicious cycle. Our children have the right to pursue their dreams without the fear of harassment or undeserved suffering.

I realize that I can't do this alone. However, with the help of committed parents, school administrators, and teachers, together we can make a tremendous impact.

I know their pain because children talk to me. Some kids look at me as some type of Super Hero that has all the answers. My philosophy is that, whatever it takes to reach our future leaders, it's alright with me. I honor their trust and use what they share with me to inform their parents of the deep challenges they face daily.

So, this book is my gift to parents and teachers with hopes of educating, inspiring, and encouraging positive change. Remember, it all starts in the home, then reinforced in the academic settings with proper care, knowledge, preparation, and execution. It's time to bring back the concept of *it takes a village to raise a child*.

Together, we WILL make a difference!

Master Samuel Scott

CHAPTER 1
WHAT IS BULLYING?

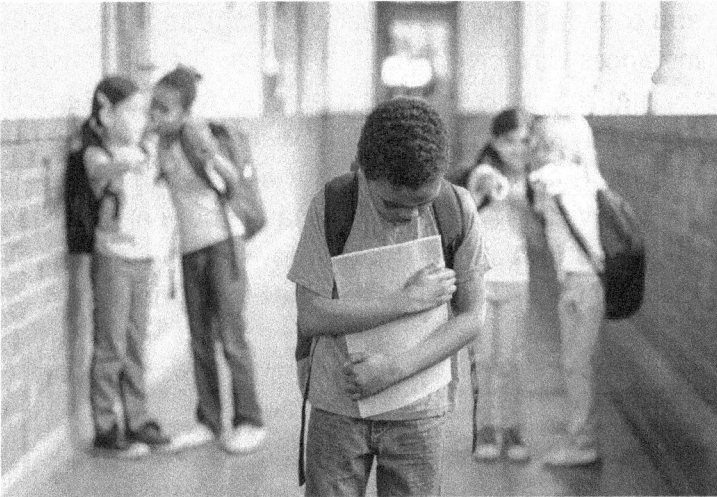

The behavior that is now known as bullying was once considered to be playground high-jinx, boys being boys, or rites of passage. Bullying is a serious abusive situation that can lead to negative, long-term issues. Bullying may not be what you think!

In fact, bullying can take on many different forms, including things like verbal harassment, physical assault, and coercion. The individual who is the aggressor in these instances is referred to as the "bully," and the victim of this aggression is referred to as the "target." Regardless of your thoughts about it or how the issues are discussed, bullying is a form of abuse. This aggression can manifest on the victim (or target) as an emotional, verbal, or physical attack and, no matter how the abuse takes place, the damage on the victim can be life-altering.

*   *   *   *   *

Hannah Smith (1999-2013). Hannah Smith, a 14-year-old girl from Lutterworth, Leicestershire, England, hanged herself in her bedroom on August 3, 2013. Her body was discovered by her older sister.

In the weeks leading up to her death, Smith had been subjected to cruel taunts and insults about her weight and a family death on Ask.fm, a question-and-answer social networking site that allows anonymous participation. Bullies on Ask.fm urged her to drink bleach and cut herself.

According to Hannah's father, she went to Ask.fm to look for advice on the skin condition eczema.

After her death, Hannah's father found a note that read: "As I sit here day by day I wonder if it's going to get better. I want to die, I want to be free. I can't live like this anymore. I'm not happy".

Following the suicide, Hannah's older sister, Jo, described how, just days after discovering her younger sister's body, she started receiving abusive messages on Facebook, mocking her loss and blaming her grieving father's parenting skills for the tragic death.

Sources: CBS, CNN and ABC News

*   *   *   *   *

Several U.S. states have enacted laws against bullying because bullying can turn into a life-long trauma for the target. Unfortunately, these laws differ vastly in their protections and guidelines as to what is considered bullying.

CHAPTER 2
TYPES OF BULLYING

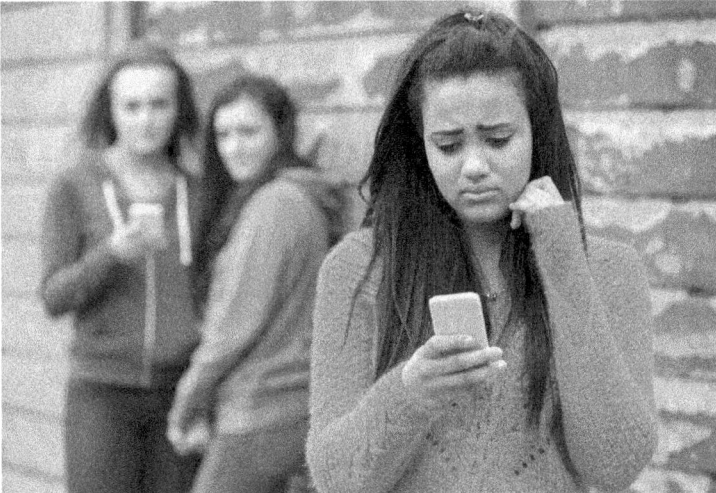

In its most basic form, bullying is the process of one person repeatedly attacking another – either with physical abuse or emotional abuse. This is a very simplistic explanation because bullying is a complex issue in which several covert ways of bullying can take place.

The U. S. National Center for Education breaks down bullying into two categories – direct and indirect:

- **Direct Bullying.** Most often direct bullying is connected to physical abuse. This includes behaviors like shoving, hitting, pulling hair, biting, pinching, punching, choking, beating, and even stabbing.

- **Indirect Bullying.** This form of bullying is more often related to emotional abuse. In this form of aggression, the bully tries to make the victim feel isolated. This is done with gossip, coercing other people to ignore or turn against the target, criticizing or teasing, laughing at the victim, spreading lies, and manipulation.

Often with indirect bullying, there is a specific reason or catalyst behind the behavior. This could be related to the perceived sexual orientation of the victim, the way one dresses, or one's race, religion, or social status.

Historically, boys were more likely to be directly bullied, and girls indirectly bullied. However, in recent years, studies have shown a change in those behaviors. Girl bullies are starting to be more aggressive and physical in their attacks, while boy bullies are starting to use exclusion more as a means of bullying.

It's true (and obvious) that one-on-one abuse can be painful for a target. What makes it even more difficult to handle is when the main bully – ring leader – pulls other people to help him with bullying. These other people are referred to as "lieutenants." (Lieutenants assist in the bullying process in which they help the bully to get away with the abusive behavior.) Lieutenants stand watch to make sure that the bully can get away with their abuse. They offer "cover-up" if the bully gets caught, and they will often join in the bullying process.

It is not clear why lieutenants are so willing to participate in bullying behavior. A few theories include:

- Maintenance of a certain social status,
- Avoidance of getting bullied, or
- The lieutenant is also a bully and enjoys making others suffer.

These theories, or none of them, could be true. However, it is important to understand that bullying isn't just something that happens on the playground or to children. Anywhere there is a human interaction, there is a potential for bullying to take place.

CHAPTER 3
THE ANATOMY OF A BULLY

/

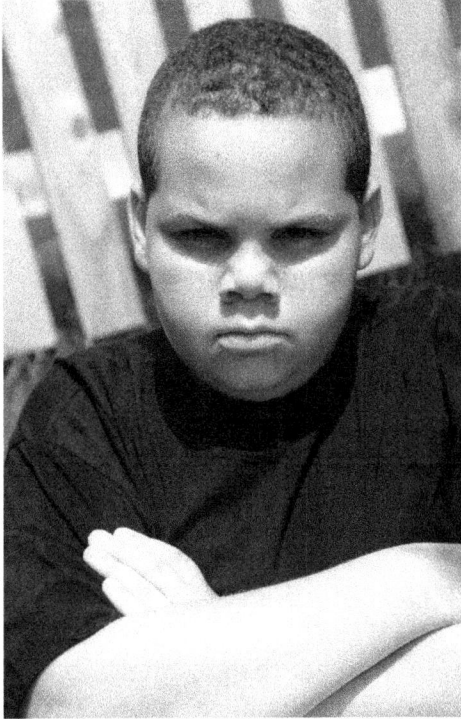

Bullies come in all shapes and sizes. There was a belief that most bullies were bigger in stature and had low self-esteem. In my school and the schools that I've visited over the years, a lot of students have openly admitted bullying bigger kids. When I asked them why they picked a child that was bigger than them, most of them said, "Because he was scared of me." This is proof that most bullies seek to control the target through fear.

In a 1978 study, Olweus characterized bullies in three different categories:

- The aggressive bully
- The passive bully
- The bully-victim

Aggressive bullies are the most common type of bully. They tend to be aggressive, hot tempered, belligerent, impulsive, confident, and physically strong. They have an aggressive personality and feed off controlling others by wielding power over them. These types of bullies tend to be looked up to and admired in their early school years.

Contrary to popular belief, these particular types of bullies do not have a self-esteem problem. They are very keen on identifying different personality traits in other kids and manipulating them.

Passive bullies, unlike the over-confident aggressive bullies, tend to be insecure with low self-esteem. They tend to have few likable qualities and a challenging home life. Passive bullies tend to be disconnected at school. Teachers have a hard time holding their attention and, as a result, they perform poorly in school. They have short tempers and exhibit violent outburst, which leads to more problems with their peers. Although they don't directly initiate bullying, they will participate in an altercation where someone is being bullied. They tend to be attracted and loyal to the more aggressive bullies.

Bully-victim is the smaller population of the three groups that have been consistent victims of bullying. They are genuinely physically weaker than those that bully them but are stronger than their own victims. They are unpopular with their peers, and in most cases, are withdrawn and depressed.

Patterns of Behavior
The following profiles fit most bullies:
- Yell and scream at targets, and most of the time in front of others.
- Criticize targets to downplay their success in front of others.
- They are excited by the conflict between others.
- Often instigate problems between two people.
- Blame others for their problems.
- Indulge in the satisfaction of others' pains, shortcomings, and fears.
- They are poor winners, boastful, self-centered, and poor losers.
- Display uncontrollable anger.
- May have a history of discipline problems at home and school.
- Display a pattern of aggressiveness.

As a result, targets that are bullied often:
- Withdraw socially and have few friends.
- Feel isolated, alone, and sad.
- Always feel like they're being picked on.
- Complain of being sick to stay home from school.

- Display mood swings, especially toward siblings.
- Feel rejected by others.
- Often display "victim" body language - drooped shoulders and sad eyes.
- Display changes in eating or sleeping habits.
- May consider taking a weapon to school for protection.

As parents, we should understand that this happens right under our noses! Therefore, it is critical that you spend quality time with your child and have open discussions about how they feel about school and friends.

CHAPTER 4
IT STARTS IN THE HOME

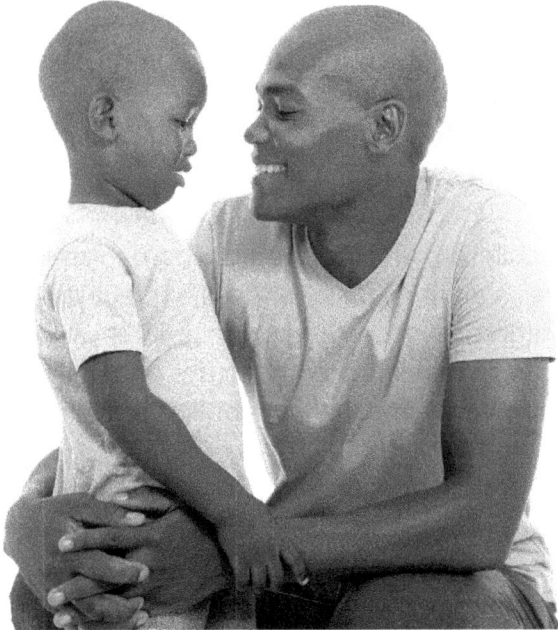

It has been proven that most bullies are simply repeating patterns of domination, power, and control that they learned from their home environments. Children who are bullied will, in turn, often bully others. This is a cycle of abuse that is difficult to stop.

In every case, bullying is a way to hold power intentionally over another individual. The reasons behind bullying are often connected to differences in class, race, religion, and sexual orientation. People who are bullied are more likely to struggle in school, have emotional problems, and even attempt suicide.

In children, antisocial traits and depression early in their lives can be clues to possible bullying in the future. Children exposed to violence in their homes are more likely to take on characteristics of a bully, and adults who bully were almost always bullies as children.

Children who once may have been accused of rough-housing or being pranksters are now being recognized as children who have the potential to bully others. These seemingly innocent playground antics can lead to much more developed systems of bullying and coercion as they grow up.

Again, if you are concerned that your child might be turning into a bully, refer to Chapter 3 under the section *Patterns of Behavior*. Often, children who bully are not taught to respect other people's feelings or to even have concern about how their actions could impact others. Behavior at home and what they are taught when they're very young can lead to bullying behavior at school-age.

Kids that bully want people to look up to them and expect others to do what they want because their caregivers have reinforced this behavior. This process starts at a very young age – before children start school. If children have no boundaries and are shown aggressive behavior from their caregivers, this teaches them that they can have whatever they want and that aggression is okay. This also teaches them to have little respect for others and creates an atmosphere where bullying will be considered acceptable to them.

When your child cannot control his or her aggression, this could be a big red flag – warning sign – that your child is headed towards becoming a bully. One of the best ways to deal with potential bullying is through counseling and teaching children how to deal with other people in a healthy and positive way.

*　　*　　*　　*　　*

Steps to help control your child's aggression

One of the ways that you can help your child in this area is by getting to the root of their anger. Often times when you drill down to get to the core issues, you'll find there is something deeper that's trigging the anger.

For example, many times at my school, when I console a child about their aggressive behavior, I quickly find out that it's usually one of the following issues:

- Lack of attention at home
- No father in the home or lack of attention from him
- Witnessed aggression in the home
- Parents divorced recently

I believe, from what I've witnessed over the years at my school, that these four challenges greatly affect a child's overall attitude.

The lack of attention at home causes a child to seek attention outside of the home. This is one of the reasons why our children turn to gangs – it gives them a sense of belonging and security.

Some of the ways I found to be most effective in handling bullying include:

- Sitting down and having an honest chat about their feelings, home life, experiences in school, friends and, of course, bullying.
- Share some of your childhood experiences as it relates to bullying (and dealing with aggressive people) because it's vital that they know you speak from experience.
- Talk about how they give the other person control over them when they become angry and aggressive.

It's crucial that you make your child feel like they can openly express themselves without feeling that they'll get ridiculed for speaking up.

Another option is to get the family involved. Most children have a favorite uncle or aunt that they feel comfortable talking with, so have them take your child out to spend some quality time. You'll be surprised to hear how they – your family member – can say the same thing to your child that you've said but get a positive response from them.

Finally, the one option that I always recommend is to enroll your child in a martial arts program that understands the needs of our young leaders. Be sure that it's a true family environment that focuses on strong character traits and life skills. Martial arts teach self-control, self-respect, and respect for others; however, having that family environment gives you another support base to help address your child's emotional needs and challenges.

*   *   *   *   *

Of course, other factors can play into the potential for a child to become a bully. Listed are some other risks:

- **School/Class Size** – Schools that have higher student populations have higher risks of bullies and victims of bullies. This is especially true when classrooms have larger student to teacher ratios. More students often mean that teachers and staff are spread thin which can give rise to more opportunities for abuse by bullies due to limited supervision.

- **Child Abuse** – Kids who have experienced abuse are 100% more likely to become a victim of bullying than kids who have not experienced abuse. Abused kids are also 50% more likely to become a bully.

- **Behavioral Issues** – Children who have a hard time expressing their feelings with words or are very shy have a higher risk of being bullied. The opposite is also true: children that cannot internalize their feeling, but aggressive at an early age, are less likely to be bullied. However, they are more likely to be the perpetrator of bullying.

Early childhood development and environmental factors in early childhood seem to be the biggest determining factor when it comes to both children that get bullied and children that become bullies. Schools that use education to teach kids about the dangers of bullying tend to have lower instances overall of bullying issues. All of the above numbers change when a school is working to teach kids not to bully.

Additionally, research has been done on adult bullies to see if their behavior started when they were children. What is known about adult bullies is that they have a need and desire to dominate others. They tend to have deeply ingrained prejudices about other people, especially those they consider "beneath" them.

Adult bullies are often authoritarian and carry deeply-seated issues around envy, jealousy, or insecurity. Self-esteem is another big factor in bullying in which many bullies have low self-esteem. Adult bullies tend to use bullying to make others seem below them which, in turn, helps them to feel better about themselves.

Studies also show that adult bullies were likely bullies as kids, especially male bullies. People that are quick to anger, have addictions, or personality disorders are more likely to bully than others. Often, bullies are tied to a specific, self-created image in which they quickly turn hostile when other's start to encroach upon their image.

CHAPTER 5
BULLYING FINALLY RECEIVING MEDIA ATTENTION

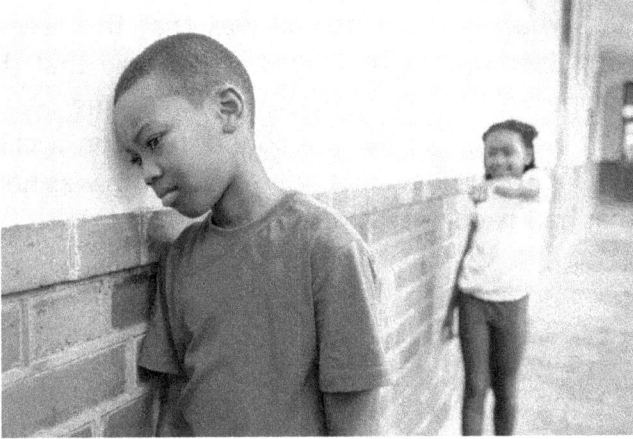

In the last few years, there have been several teenage suicides connected to bullying. These tragic deaths have prompted several movements about bullying awareness. Though many of these suicides were related to a teenager's sexual orientation, this was not true for all of them.

Yet, what was true for all was that the teens felt so ostracized and alone that they believed that their only escape was to kill themselves. It has long been known that bullying can have serious effects on a child, even leading to suicide. Yet, until recently, this was not an area that had been greatly researched.

*   *   *   *   *

In 1999, when the Columbine High School shootings took place in Littleton, CO, this was the first in a series of school shootings where it was later revealed that the killers felt this was the only way to get revenge on their bullies and to end their suffering.

With the Columbine tragedy, two teenage boys killed 13 people and wounded 24 others before they each committed suicide. After the Columbine information came out, it was learned that the two boys, who were considered gifted students, had been bullied by their classmates for years. These boys took months to play out the attack in which they wrote long stories about why they were going to murder all the kids that had made their lives so hard. The two used the shootings as a way of getting back on the society that they believed *had turned against them, seeing no other way but to end their lives.*

*   *   *   *   *

Following Columbine, there have been a series of other school shootings across the United States. Unfortunately, these types of terror acts happen every school year and, most often, the children involved in the violence are acting out of a need to seek revenge on the school – the bullies – that made their lives unbearable for so long.

After several school shootings took place, the U.S. Secret Service released an analysis showing that, in two-thirds of the school shootings, the attackers had been bullied. In interviews after the attacks, some of the school shooters even described their time in school as torment. Often, the kids that are bullied are considered gifted students (or do well in school).

School officials often ignore bullying, and even some of the victims try to ignore the abusive behavior by not reporting the abuse or by attempting to avoid the bullies on their own. In many cases, ignoring the behavior gives rise to the victims being bullied more, especially when they don't report it to teachers or parents.

With school-age children, bullying can happen in the classroom, but it is much more likely to take place in areas where adult supervision is light or non-existent. You will find that kids are bullied during recess, between classes, in the bathroom, on the school bus, or in after-school activities more so than in class.

*   *   *   *   *

My Childhood Experience with Bullying

Although I spent the last 25 years researching and teaching about this growing epidemic, it's important to know that growing up I, too, was a victim of bullying.

Growing up in a tough neighborhood in Long Island, NY, called Gordon Heights, you had to know how to defend yourself just to get on the school bus or to go to the neighborhood park.

As an athletic, middle-school student – sixth grader – I decided to join the wrestling team. During that time, my only motivation was to learn how to protect myself better against the older boys in our school. Most of the boys on the wrestling team were eighth graders, but because of my size I was allowed to train with them.

For the most part, the guys on the team were pretty cool. I mean they loved tossing the newbie sixth grader around the mat like a rag doll. After a while, they all respected the fact that I was a fierce competitor and they accepted me as one of the guys.

However, there was this one kid, who was an eighth grader, that literally hated my very presence in the locker room. On some occasions, for no reason at all, he would just walk up and shove me in my chest. Having a phobia about the "big tough eighth graders," I froze up every time. This went on for maybe two weeks or more. At first, I thought that the aggression towards me from this bully would just eventually go away; instead, he became more and more aggressive.

I remember leaving practice each day upset with myself for letting this kid bully me. As a result of this constant bullying, I found myself lashing out at my siblings, not wanting to go to the neighborhood park and, at times, not wanting to eat dinner with my family.

One day, I woke up and said to myself, "That's the last time that he puts his hands on me." Back in those days, there were no bully prevention programs, and you surely didn't tell your teacher about it – that was completely off limits. Was I afraid? Absolutely! However, something inside of me said, "Stand up to this bully once and for all!" On the day I decided to stand up, as I was walking to shop class, our paths crossed. He was walking with his girlfriend and gesturing to me as if to say, "There's the coward right there." She looked at me and smiled. Right when we were about to pass each other, I turned and shoved him. He looked at me in total shock – it was on!

We fought like cats and dogs. I was so angry that I completely overwhelmed him physically. When the teacher came over to break us up, he swung and knocked his glasses off, breaking them in half. The two of us were sent to the office and, as I looked over at him, he looked like a little puppy. The once big, bad wolf turned out to be nothing more than a coward that wanted to dominate and control weaker kids.

Eventually, he admitted to the principal that he was, in fact, harassing me during wrestling practice. He also admitted to breaking the teacher's glasses. In the end, he sincerely apologized to me and, for the rest of my middle and high school experience, he was nothing short of pleasant and respectful.

Now, let's be clear: I'm not encouraging or alluding to the fact that kids should go out and start fighting bullies. However, what I am saying is that, contrary to the advice of the so-called experts, running and telling a teacher or parent or asking him to stop or to be his friend, doesn't always solve the bully issue.

Yes, I absolutely support and promote the different progressive steps as it relates to addressing the bully problem. However, as a last resort, standing up and asserting yourself not only lets the bully know that you can and will defend yourself, but it also alerts and puts other bullies and bystanders on notice as well.

In the real world, it's called earning your respect.

*   *   *   *   *

A study from the Archives of General Psychiatry studied data from a 1981 Finish Birth Cohort study. The researchers took 5,813 children that were born in Finland in 1981 and collected data on their psychiatric symptoms at the age of eight. They then followed these same children through ages 13 to 24. The goal of this study was to determine if children, who were expressing bullying behavior at the age of eight, would have psychiatric issues as they got older.

The study put the children into four different classification groups based on their bullying behavior when they were eight years old. The first group – or #1 – was comprised of children who were never victims or bullies. The second group – or #2 – was made up of children who were bullies only. The third group – or #3 – were children who were victims of bullying only. The final group – or #4 – were children who were both victims of bullying and bullies.

What they discovered was split between girls and boys.
The females that were victims of bullying, but never bully themselves, had much higher risks for later psychiatric issues and psychiatric medication. When they checked at the age of eight for psychiatric symptoms that could lead to these issues, they discovered that these children were not on track to have issues into adulthood with psychiatric problems.

The males had a higher risk for future psychiatric issues anytime they were a victim of bullying, even if they later became bullies themselves. But at the age of eight, these boys were on track to have psychiatric issues later in life.

So, were the boys in this study picked on because they were different or did their being bullied lead to their later psychological issues? It's hard to say, but what is clear is that bullying can cause emotional and psychological problems well into adulthood

*   *   *   *   *

Shocking Truth from My Students that Totally Shocked Their Parents

One day, I decided to surprise my young students by teaching their class, and the school was packed with students and parents. I had the instructors warm up the class, before I walked on the floor. The students were looking at me as if they just saw a ghost. I started teaching, and the kids and parents were having an awesome time.

Close to the end of class, I sat the students down for what I thought was going to be a quick "mat chat."

I started out by praising them for doing an awesome job in class and being so attentive and focused. Then I started talking to them about bullying. Immediately, the mood changed! It was so quiet that you could hear a pin drop. Their body language made it evident that many of them had been victims of bullying or was a bully themselves.

I remember taking a deep breath and saying, "I would like for us to have a family chat. For the moment, I want you to act as though no one here is listening to us. I want you to be very honest with your answers so that we can do our best to address any challenges that some of you may have."

The first question I asked was, "How many of you have been bullied at school or in the neighborhood?" To our surprise, over 95% of the kids put their hands up. Now keep in mind, we are talking about kids between the ages of 7 and 13 years old. You could hear a deep gasp from the parents as they looked at each other in total shock. Next, I asked, "How many of you witnessed someone else being bullied?" Again about 95% of them raised their hands. I then asked, "How many of you were, at one point or another, a bully yourself?"

About 20% of the room put their hands up. I thanked them for their honest confession as most kids would never admit being a bully. Finally, I asked the most important question: "How many of you actually told your parents or teachers about the incidents?" Nearly 80% said that they didn't tell anyone! Many of the parents were totally caught off guard, thinking that they had a good relationship with their child.

I then asked some of the kids to stand up and share their stories. All I can say is that there wasn't a dry eye in the building. They told their stories of how kids were teasing them all day long. How they were being pushed around in the hallways and on the school bus. One kid talked about how he was ganged up on in the bathroom by three boys.

Of all the stories, there was one that caused everyone in the building to shed tears. It was told by a little six-year-old girl who appeared to be one of the bubbliest kids in our school. She shared how this big girl in her class would call her names and pull her hair. As she told her story, you could see and feel just how hurt she was from it all. I asked her, "How did it make you feel?" She replied, "Sad, very sad." I asked her, "Did you tell the teacher?" She said, "Yes, but the girl kept on pulling my hair every day." She also said that she didn't tell her parents because she thought she would get in trouble for fighting.

This one session prompted us to re-implement our Bully Busting Program. We made a mistake thinking that, because they were super happy kids that always walk in with big smiles on their faces, they weren't victims of bullying.

The great news is that they trusted us, their martial arts family, enough to share their inner thoughts and feelings. Who knows what could've happened if many of these kids continued to hide what was happening to them on a daily basis? This is why it is so important to speak to your child about the bully problem. More importantly, as mentioned, you have to know the signs and indicators of potential bullying so that you can catch it early. Lastly, never underestimate the power of a mentor – that person just might be the person that your child will share their feelings.

As the old saying goes, "It takes a village to raise a child."

*   *   *   *   *

CHAPTER 6
IS MY CHILD A BULLY?

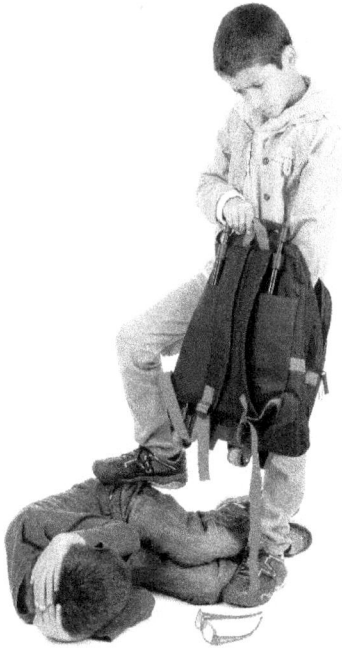

Too often, parents brush aside any concerns that they might have about their own children being potential bullies. Some tend to think bullying others and getting bullied is just a natural part of growing up, but it isn't. If you are concerned that your child might be a bully, you need to treat this very seriously.

Don't just trust what your child is telling you. Kids are amazingly skilled at manipulating adults, especially their parents. They might tell you the truth that they want you to hear and spin the information from a perspective where they look innocent. It is better to talk to their teacher to find out what may really be going on.

This is a fact that can be hard for many parents to accept. You don't want to think that your child could be bullying other children because you want to trust what they tell you and maintain a good relationship with them. This is important, but you need to make sure that their behavior matches the values that you are trying to instill in them by investigating your instincts or the comments told you by others regarding your child.

It can be hard to accept that your child is behaving like a bully, however, dealing with it is better than ignoring it and allowing the abusive behavior. Besides, abusive behavior – bullying – is illegal.

Most likely, the victim of your child's bullying or the school is keeping a record of the events that have been taking place. Pay attention to those reports! Is there a pattern that you can discern from what is happening in your child's home life that might be connected to the time or days that they have been accused of bullying others?

Often there is something happening in the home environment of a bullying child that causes them to act out aggressively. Examine your home life and ask some tough questions:

- Could there be reasons for your child's aggression?
- Is it possible that your child might have a disorder that needs to be addressed with professional help?

These can be heartbreaking questions to answer for any parent but ignoring the issue will only make it worse for your child and you in the long term.

*   *   *   *   *

I grew up in New York with a close friend whom I'll call "Frank." When we were about 13 years old, at least once a week when I was at his home, it seemed like his parents were always arguing and fighting. On several occasions, I remember looking at my friend and seeing his eyes gleaming with anger. He never really talked about what he was feeling, but you could tell that it was getting to him. Later, when he started dating, I noticed that he would get angry with his girlfriends for the slightest thing.

While at a party one day, Frank got mad because his girlfriend was dancing with another one of our friends. He walked up to her, started yelling at her, and then shoved her. I immediately stepped in front of her and asked him, "What is your problem?" He looked at me and then stormed out of the party.

The next day, I went to Frank's house to talk to him, and he was very apologetic. It was as if he were another person. I asked him what was bothering him, he replied, "I don't know, it seems like I can't control my anger."

Sad to say that my friend grew up and became a violent abuser. He started drinking and turning to drugs. The violent environment as a child eventually took its toll on Frank. He has spent most of his adult life in and out of jail for domestic violence.

*   *   *   *   *

No matter what, you must remember that your child is responsible for his actions. You should be clear with your child that you will not allow bullying behavior. You should express that all bullying activities must stop immediately, and that you will be checking on them to make sure that they are following your orders.

Remember, you are the adult, and you are the one in charge. Be strong and firm, but also be mindful that you don't border on bullying since this can be a very confusing message for your child to understand.

Once you have a clear idea that abuse is happening, it is now your job as a parent to help your child change their behavior and stop the cycle of abuse. Though this can be a difficult process, here are some helpful steps to modify the behavior when your child has been acting like a bully:

- **Set the Rules.** Create house and family rules. It is important that you reinforce these rules with rewards when things are done as you required. Rewarding positive behavior is much more effective than punishing negative behavior. Punishment usually doesn't work but, if rules continue to be broken, the best form of punishment is to take away privileges – like computer access, cell phone, or television time.

- **Spend Time Together.** It could be that your child is bullying as a means of acting out for your attention. Spending more time with your child will not only help to change the negative behavior, but it will also help you to monitor their behavior in different situations more easily.

- **Check on Their Friends.** Your child may be associated with kids that are encouraging their bullying behavior. Take time to meet your child's friends and get to know them. This can help you to determine if certain friendships instigate their bullying behavior. If their friends seem to be a bad influence, encourage them to forge friendship with other kids, limit their access to these children, and get them involved with after-school activities away from these kids.

- **Reward Positive Behavior.** By celebrating when your child is exhibiting positive traits, you help to reinforce more of that behavior. In a short amount of time, you will see that their behavior becomes kinder and less aggressive.

CHAPTER 7
BYSTANDERS (A GROWING PROBLEM IN THIS COUNTRY)

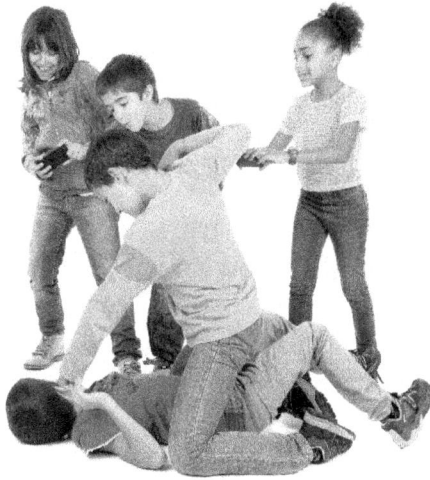

A main problem with bullying is the fact that so many people, both children and adults, stand by and watch it happen. Usually, there are witnesses to acts of bullying, but these witnesses do not stop the process, intercede, or do anything to help the victims. If the bully isn't challenged by bystanders or stopped, this only reinforces the negative behavior and helps to create a stronger bully.

Often, bystanders don't intervene in these situations as an act of self-preservation which is especially true with children. The thought process is that, if the bully's attention is on someone else, that child can avoid being bullied themselves. This is the exact behavior a bully needs to continue to gain power.

Another way that bystanders reinforce the abusive behavior is by joining in the activities that the bully is doing. Bystanders will often get involved with the bullying by either teasing the victim themselves or encouraging the bully to continue with their abusive behavior. This is another process of deflection by taking the attention away from themselves and keeping it on the target of the bullying.

Bullies love to have people watching them and, if a bystander steps in and expresses displeasure in what is taking place, the bullying will often stop. It can take a real act of courage to step in and stop bullying from happening, but it can be very powerful.

*   *   *   *   *

Recently while viewing my Facebook page, I saw a post about a child being bullied by a bigger kid while other students stood by and watched. Instead of intervening, kids were laughing, and some literally had their phones out videotaping the incident. The teacher stood by, and you could hardly hear her saying anything to stop the attack.

Fed up with being pushed around by this much bigger kid and with no one willing to step in and help, the victim fought back and completely overwhelmed the bully. Again, we don't advocate fighting. However, when your child's back is against the wall, they must defend themselves to avoid serious injury.

*   *   *   *   *

Now, if your child comes home and tells you that they have been a bullying bystander and they are witnessing abuse that is happening at their school, you have an important opportunity to have a conversation about bullying and what they can do to potentially stop it, including reporting it to school authorities.

Here are some suggestions that you can offer your child as a witness (or bystander) the next time a bully starts their abuse:

- **Walk Away**. When you take away a bully's audience, often the bullying stops. Encourage your child to walk away and see if they can get other kids to walk away with them, including the child that is being bullied.

- **Speak Up.** If your child tells a bully to stop or tells them what they are doing isn't funny, they are more likely to stop the abuse. Once one child stands up to a bully, it makes it easier for the other kids to do the same.

- **Ask for Help.** Many times, kids won't go to an adult or ask for help because they are worried this will get them into trouble or lead to their being bullied. Yet, by getting adult intervention, the bully knows that they can't get away with their behavior. Once an adult knows what is going on, that child will be watched more closely.

- **Offer Friendship.** Sometimes bullies will go after kids that don't have a lot of friends because they think they are easy targets. If your child offers that child friendship, it will make it harder for the bully to single them out.

Once you hear from your child that there is bullying happening, even if it isn't happening to them, you really should report it. Talk to your child's teacher and the school administrators – the school needs to know what is going on within their school because they are responsible for each child inside their doors.

It's also a good idea to occasionally check back with the school to see how things are going with the situation and to determine if there has been any resolution.

Responsibility
Many people look at continual bullying as solely the responsibility of the bully but, in order for this bullying to continue, there must be some amount of responsibility placed on the victim. The bully will only continue to be abusive if they can do so. For bullying to stop, the victim must make it clear that they will no longer tolerate the abusive behavior. Granted, this is often easier said than done.

Changing a bully's behavior can happen through several means.

- **Turning the Action.** When a victim of bullying turns the action, they change the target of the behavior from themselves back to the bully. This makes the victim become the bully, and the bully becomes the victim.

- **Conversation.** It is possible to talk to the bully and diffuse the attacks. When the victim becomes real to the bully and not just a target, it is harder for the bully to continue to be abusive.

- **Telling.** Reporting the behavior to an authority figure can stop bullying, but this doesn't always work. Occasionally "tattle-telling" only leads to more abuse and bullying. However, in order to have the behavior monitored, it is important to report what is happening.

- **Legal Intervention.** When the complaints and reporting don't help to stop the behavior, taking legal action can show that the victim is serious and won't accept the abuse any longer.

The reason that certain people tend to be repeatedly bullied in their lives is because they unknowingly position themselves to be a target. For instance, people that don't react well to stress or stand up for themselves are more likely to be marked by a bully. This is not to say that it is the target's fault but working on the self-esteem and confidence of a target can help the behavior to stop.

For bullying to work, there must be an act of submission that happens after the act of aggression. If the victim does not offer the submission, then the bully's behavior cannot be successful and less likely to attempt that behavior with that same target. It is most effective to break this cycle at the first attempt of bullying. Even after years of abuse, the cycle can still be broken but not as easily.

CHAPTER 8
CYBER BULLYING

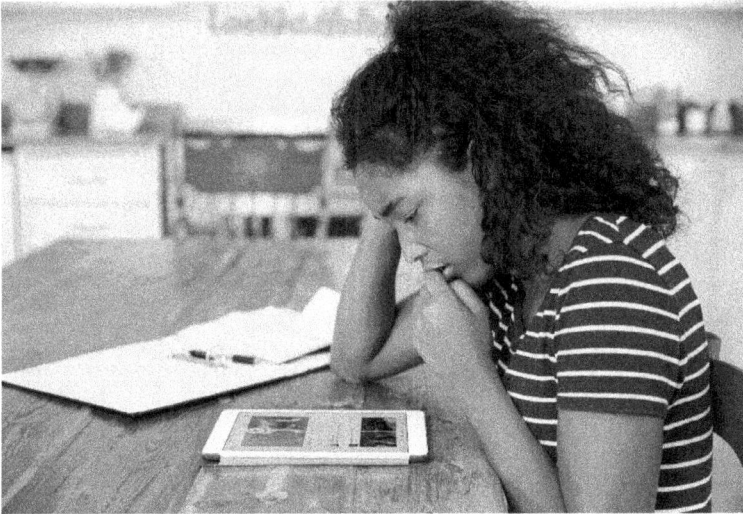

Cyberbullying is growing in use, especially among young people. Cyberbullying is the practice of using the internet and social media to bully another person, often anonymously. This can happen through email, instant messaging, texting, and other means of social networking. Since you can pose as anyone online, it is difficult to catch the perpetrators of cyberbullying.

Cyber-stalking, another more specific form of cyber-harassment and acts of sexual predation, is not considered cyberbullying. Cyberbullying is connected to a very specific set of acts with a particular desired outcome. It is not uncommon for kids to communicate with their friends through electronic mediums with lewd or aggressive language but, again, it is not considered a form of cyberbullying.

Typically, cyberbullying doesn't happen as a one-time occurrence. For behavior to be considered cyberbullying, it would have to take place over a period and be a series of habitual harassment through electronic means. True cyberbullying goes way beyond sending a dirty message or aggressive language.

Sometimes hacking is involved in cyberbullying. In these instances, the bully hacks into the email or social media accounts of the victim and sends messages as if they were sent from the victim. These messages are often damaging to social status, friendships, romantic partnerships, and family. This form of cyberbullying is a serious criminal offense in both state and federal laws.

Schools are highly ineffective when it comes to cyberbullying because the bullying usually doesn't happen on school grounds or where they have jurisdiction.

*   *   *   *   *

Phoebe Prince. *Phoebe Prince was a 15-year-old Irish immigrant, a student at South Hadley High School in Massachusetts. Pheobe hanged herself two days before the winter cotillion dance at her school. Pheobe, a newcomer to the school, was a victim of cyberbullying about her date for that dance, a senior football player.*

Phoebe was subjected to an onslaught of bullying and was called "Irish slut" and "whore" on Twitter, Craigslist, Facebook and Formspring, and in person at the school. Even after her death, the girls left vicious messages on a Facebook page created in her memory.

Sources: CBS, CNN and ABC News

*   *   *   *   *

What schools can do is to educate students on how the dangers of cyberbullying. Many schools offer trainings, workshops, and presentations on bullying and adding cyberbullying as part of that conversation has proven to be highly effective.

Recent studies show that cyberbullying affects close to half of all American teenagers. In 2006, an ABC News report showed that out of 1,500 kids, between the fourth through eighth grades, experienced the following instances of cyberbullying:

- 42% of the kids felt that they had been bullied online and one in four had it happen more than one time.

- 35% of the kids felt threatened while online and one in five had it happen more than one time.

- 21% of the kids had received mean or threatening messages.

- 58% of the kids had someone say mean or hurtful things about them online and more than four out of ten had this happen more than once.

- 58% of the kids never told anyone what happened to them with this abuse while online.

Kids who experienced cyberbullying expressed the same responses that would be expected from kids who are bullied in person. Things like skipping school, running away, and abuse of drugs and alcohol were experienced with both groups.

It is hard to monitor cyberbullying, but it is no less damaging to a person. This is a growing area of bullying as more and more people spend their time communicating online.

CHAPTER 9
CYBER BULLYING VS. TRADITIONAL BULLYING

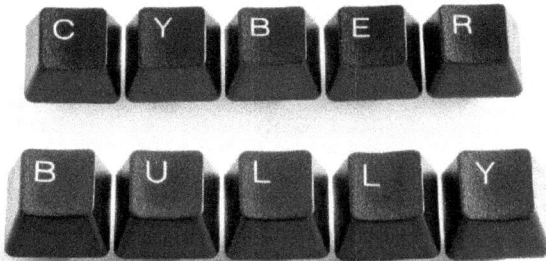

There are many similarities between cyberbullying and traditional person-to-person bullying, but there are also many differences. The most obvious difference is that face-to-face bullying always has the potential to get physically violent, but there are also many other factors that make cyberbullying such a scary prospect.

The internet makes it easy for cyber bullies to remain anonymous. By using temporary accounts or fake names, these bullies can continue to harass their targets for as long as they want to without any of the constraints that might be felt from face-to-face or traditional bullying methods. Cyberbullying provides the bully with the freedom to act out in ways that they would never have the courage to do in front of witnesses.

Most social networking sites and chat rooms have no supervision. For the most part, when someone is in a chat room, they can post whatever they want and there's very little regulation to do anything about it. Many times, parents of bullied teens are unable to help. Often kids and teens know more about internet functions than their parents which only helps to mask potentially negative behaviors.

What is most difficult about cyberbullying versus traditional bullying methods is the lack of safety. With traditional bullying, the victim always has a place to go where they can escape the bullying – usually home. With cyberbullying, the safety and security of the home is broken because the cyber-attacks follow them into their safe places.

This type of intrusiveness leaves the targets feeling vulnerable, nullifying any real sense of privacy or security anywhere they go. It can be extremely isolating, even more so than traditional bullying. Cyberbullying is much harder to stop. Even if the bullies stop posting defamatory material, once posted, it is nearly impossible to eliminate the material online.

Millions of people could have already seen, printed, and reposted the information that the bullies put online. Pictures of the victim can be posted and edited to make it look like they have participated in certain undesirable events.

There have been several reports of young teenage girls having nude or pornographic pictures posted online. These girls didn't pose for these pictures but were the victims of photo doctoring. Even when the original posting has been removed, these doctored photos can still be on the internet.

*   *   *   *   *

Story about a 10-year old that Committed Suicide

As I began to bring this book to a close, a frightening news flash came across my computer:

10-year old Ashawnty Davis committed suicide over a video of a fight with an alleged bully.

According to her parents, Ashawnty, a sixth grader, was a happy girl who had aspirations of becoming a star basketball player. The parents stated that, in October, all of that changed after a video of her fight was put on social media. The video showed Ashawnty and another girl fighting while the other students watched.

The Father said that, *"She was devastated when she found out that it had made it to Musical.Ly. My daughter came home two weeks later and hung herself in her closet."*
She was on life support for two weeks at Children's Hospital in Colorado before passing away Wednesday morning, November 29th.

The Father said, *"That was my baby, and I love my baby, and I just want mothers to listen."*

*   *   *   *   *

This tragedy struck me at the core as all I could do is think about my daughter. As parents, we work so hard to protect our babies, inspiring and encouraging them to be the best that they can be and, in a blink of an eye, a bully can come along and literally drive our children to commit suicide. It's devastatingly unfair to the parents and family members who have to spend the rest of their lives with memories of the tragic loss of their babies.

We must put an end to this growing epidemic before it's too late.

On the other hand, victims can avoid the bullying by not visiting the websites or chat rooms where the bullying is taking place. If the bullies cannot get a reaction from the victim, they are less likely to continue with the abusive behavior. In certain social networking sites, people can be blocked or filtered. This system of blocking and filtering can help to prevent some of the harassment from cyberbullying.

Several states in the U.S. have laws against cyberbullying. A federal law is in the works – but not yet existent – which is why states are putting them into effect. California was the first state to pass laws dealing with cyberbullying. Their law gives power to school administrators to discipline students both offline and online.

CHAPTER 10
HOW TO TELL IF YOUR CHILD IS BEING BULLIED

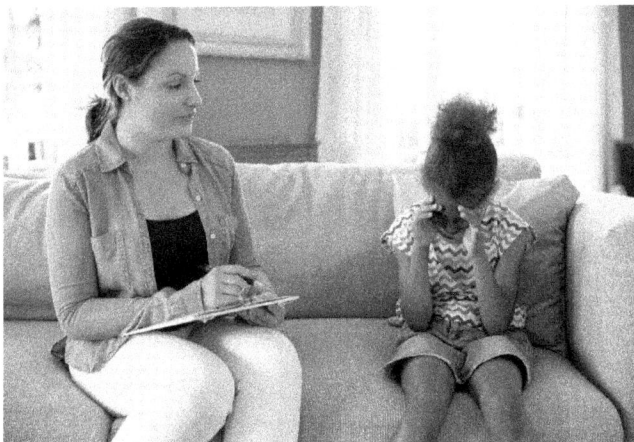

Most of the time when a child is being bullied, they aren't going to just come and tell you that they are being teased or tormented. They are going to act out in other ways that say things to hint that something is wrong. As their parent, it is up to you to pick up on signals that indicate that something is not right.

Look for changes in the child. However, be aware that not all children who are bullied exhibit warning signs. Here are some of the most common clues that something isn't right with your child and their school situation: (Source: Stopbullying.gov)

- If your child always loved going to school and suddenly doesn't want to go anymore, this is a big red flag. If they pretend to be sick or have other excuses for not going to school, it is a good time to start asking probing questions.
- Unexplainable injuries.
- Lost or destroyed clothing, books, electronics, or jewelry.
- Frequent headaches or stomach aches, feeling sick or faking illness.
- Changes in eating habits, like suddenly skipping meals or binge eating. Kids may come home from school hungry because they did not eat lunch.
- Difficulty sleeping or frequent nightmares.
- Declining grades, loss of interest in schoolwork, or not wanting to go to school.
- Sudden loss of friends or avoidance of social situations.
- Feelings of helplessness or decreased self-esteem.

- Self-destructive behaviors such as running away from home, harming themselves, or talking about suicide.

*   *   *   *   *

Bullying Almost Ruins Child's Straight "A" Record

About a year after opening our martial arts school, a parent walked into my office with tears in her eyes asking if I could please talk to her son about his grades. I was totally taken by surprise as this young man, who I'll call Robert, had for years been consistently on the Honor Roll list. He was the kid that was always on our Academic Achievers' list at our martial arts school as well. I asked her what was going on with him. She stated that she had no idea, he just went from Honor Roll to C's and D's. Now, keep in mind, that he was in the seventh grade, so he was well adjusted to the middle school academic level.

The next day she brought Robert into my office and, immediately, his body language told me that something was deeply troubling him. He had very sad eyes, drooped shoulders, low energy, and hardly any eye contact. I went into the file cabinet and pulled out all of his prior report cards and certificates that he had turned in over the years. (He was shocked that we even kept them!) As I began to remind him about those proud moments of how he used to come running into the school with his report card waving in the air, he cracked a smile and, for a minute, he seemed like his old self again.

After spending some time taking him down memory lane, I asked Robert, "What happened?" He looked down, then looked at his mom and started to cry. I told him that it was alright to cry and to take his time. When he finally got himself together, he mumbled that he was being picked on and bullied all day in school. He said the kids were teasing him, calling him the teacher's pet, nerd, and goofball. He said it started out with two kids and grew to about eight kids. He said to me, "They were everywhere! In my class, in the gym, outside during rec time and on the bus." He stated that he hated when the teacher would call his name out for getting a hundred on his class test because, as soon as they left the class, the teasing would start.

His mom was shocked! She said, "This is the first I'm hearing this." She yelled at him saying, "Why didn't you tell me ... why didn't you say something?" Robert just looked down and continued to cry.

Now, I want to add that Robert's parents had very demanding jobs which required them to work long hours. The father traveled a lot, so he wasn't home to give his son the support he needed.

After listening to Robert share his horrifying story, I thanked him for being honest and trusting me enough to confide in me. Then I went to work to try to get him back on track with his academic gift. I shared with him how I, too, was a victim of bullying. He looked at me in total amazement. I told him that it got so bad that I didn't want to go to school anymore. I told him how I made the same mistake of not telling anyone – I just kept it to myself. I said, "Then one day, I made a decision not to allow anyone to bully me again." I told him how I stood up against the bully and how that ended my days of being a victim of bullying. My message to him was that it was my decision to no longer be a victim of bullying.

I then looked him in the eyes and said, "You now have to make that decision for yourself young leader. There are kids in your school and neighborhood that don't want anything out of life. They want you, and other young bright leaders, to be like them – losers. It's a choice that they've made and, believe me, they are going to get exactly what they put out there in the world.

You, on the other hand, made the decision a long time ago to travel the path of a leader. That's why you were so focused in school and here during your martial arts training. Don't let these bad kids destroy your future. You are a bright, handsome and strong future leader, and life will reward you for your hard work." I closed the meeting by telling him that we had his back, and we were going to come to his school to visit him. He was full of joy and super excited about our talk and my commitment to him.

Afterward, I spoke privately with his mother. Before I could say anything, she literally broke down in tears, thanking me for being there for her and her child. I took this opportunity to encourage her, as humbly as I possibly could, to spend more time with him. I asked her to make him feel that it's okay to talk to you about his challenges. Lastly, I encouraged her to visit his school and to get to know his teachers as well as the admin staff. "Let them see that you are a concerned and supportive parent." She received it well and went on to do just that.

The next quarter, Robert was back on the Honor Roll and has since gone on to graduate high school and college with honors. He is now an engineer just like his Father.

*   *   *   *   *

CHAPTER 11
LONG-TERM EFFECTS OF BULLYING

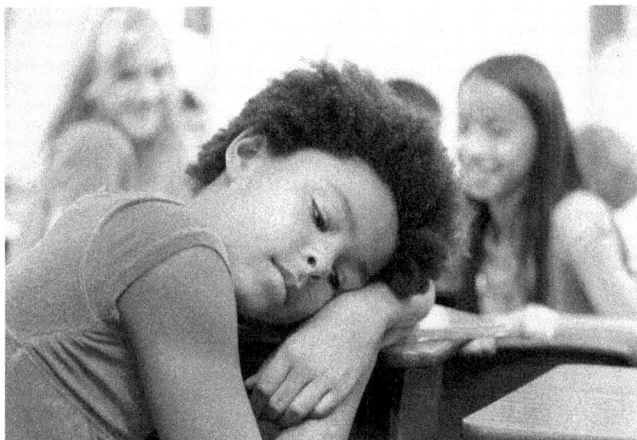

You might think that only the targets of bullying will have the potential for long-term issues, but the reality is that the bully, the victim, and bystanders of bullying can have long-term psychological issues related to the bullying events.

Victims of bullying, or targets, will typically have poor psychosocial adjustment. They are typically singled out for being different, and it is unclear from the studies on bullying if being different causes bullying or if bullying further causes differences.

Kids who are bullied tend to have a hard time making friends and might be socially awkward. Since they feel alone, they are more likely to skip school to avoid the bullying behavior. They are also more likely to use drugs and alcohol as a means of numbing their pain.

Later in life, targets of bullying are more likely to have depression in adulthood and are at a higher risk for suicide. Some studies have also shown that kids who experienced bullying against them as children were twice as likely to have psychotic symptoms develop during adolescence.

Although the kids that are bullies have fewer long-term issues, they by no means escape without any issues at all. A high percentage of school bullies end up being the perpetrators of serious crimes as they move towards adulthood. They are also at a higher risk for smoking and alcohol abuse.

People who are bystanders to bullying often suffer from fear during the events. This is because they feel that they could be the next victim of the abusive behavior.

Typically, long-term issues are not as much of a problem for bystanders; however, preventing bullying is possible by working with bystanders to stop the negative behavior.

CHAPTER 12
BULLY RELATED SUICIDE OR BULLYCIDE

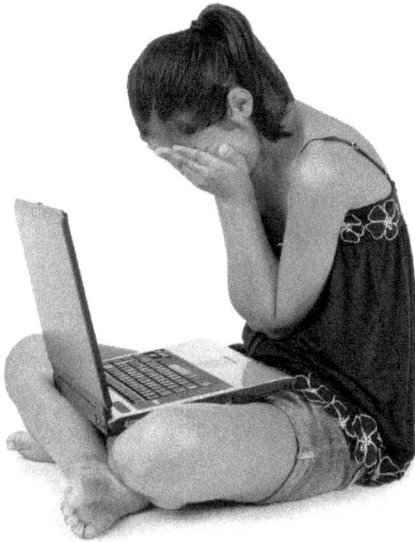

Did you know that the leading cause of death for children under 14 years of age is suicide? In a recent study from the Yale School of Medicine that review the deaths of young people in over 13 countries, there was a connection between being bullied and suicide. This is the ultimate response to being bullied and one of the most heartbreaking responses.

What makes these numbers scarier is that they are on the rise, and the ages of children turning to suicide to end their pain is getting younger. This is not to say that all children who experience bullying will head down a road of depression that ends with suicide, but children that are bullied are more likely to take their own lives – a fact that cannot be disputed.

The term *bullycide*, which is used to describe people who have killed themselves rather than deal with the continual abuse and bullying that they were receiving from their peers, was coined in 2001 in the book *Bullycide: Death at Playtime*. In the last few years, this term has become more well-known due to a string of very public teen suicides in response to cyberbullying attacks.

The public outcry against bullying and teen suicide due to bullying developed an online event called Spirit Day. On this day, people wear purple to show their support to those that have been bullied and to represent their opposition to bullying. The majority of this has come from the LGBTQ communities.

Children who identify as lesbian, gay, bisexual, transgendered, or questioning have even higher rates of abuse, bullying, and suicide. In 2007, a study by the Gay, Lesbian, and Straight Education Network, or GLSEN, found that 86 percent of LGBTQ students had experienced some form of bullying or harassment regarding their sexual orientation.

*   *   *   *   *

__Kenneth Weishuhn, Jr.__ (1997-2012). Kenneth Weishuhn, a gay high school freshman from Paullina, Iowa, took his own life after being bullied by classmates at school and online, and with death threats by phone.

The bullying began with an anti-gay Facebook group, created by Kenneth's classmates. His mother, Jeannie Chambers, said she knew her son was being harassed, and said that her son told her, "Mom, you don't know how it feels to be hated."

According to his sister Kayla, the abuse that started after he "came out" was from people he had trusted: "People that were originally his friends, they kind of turned on him. A lot of people, they either joined in or were too scared to say anything."

Sources: CBS, CNN and ABC News

*   *   *   *   *

Their research goes on to report that LGBTQ children are twice as likely to attempt suicide as their counterparts. Here are some statistics about the bullying of LGBTQ youth:

- Half of all youth said they had been physically harassed.

- A quarter had been physically assaulted.

- 9 out of 10 had been harassed verbally specifically related to their sexual orientation.

- Two-thirds of these students didn't report the harassment and, when they did, one-third of them received no support from school staff.

CHAPTER 13
WHAT TO DO ABOUT BULLYING

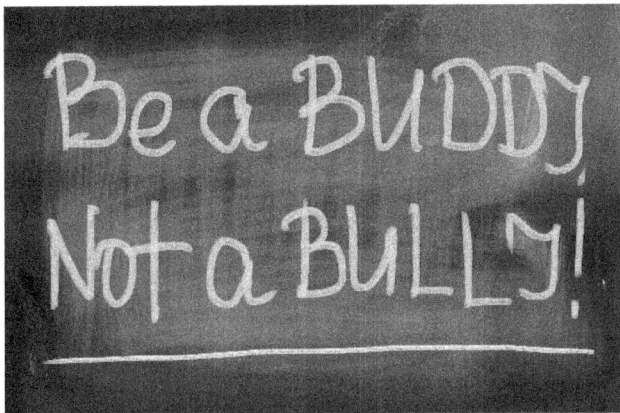

If you have reason to believe that your child is being bullied at school, there are several things that you can do. These things can be done with or without your child's knowledge, so it is best to act as soon as you start to have concerns about changes in their behavior.

If you believe that your child is being bullied and they won't talk to you about it, the best thing to do is talk to their teacher first. Do this before school starts by setting up an appointment or sending an email to meet with an administrator.

Kids are very sneaky when it comes to bullying. Your child is not going to be bullied in front of the teacher. Don't be quick to blame the teacher for not paying attention, since the bullying might not be happening when they are around, and they can't be around all the time. Also, don't expect that the school already knows that this behavior is happening. Most likely, if they knew, they would have informed you.

When you go to talk to your child's teacher, remember that you are asking for their help. You are asking them to keep an eye out for strange or inappropriate behavior. You can then follow-up to see if they uncovered bullying behavior.

If the teacher doesn't discover anything and you know that something is still happening, you can take it to the next step and meet with the principal. If your child tells you that they are being bullied, it is important that they feel supported by you. Some of the worst, unsupportive things that you can do:

- Is to ask your child, 'what they did to deserve the teasing?'
- Tell them, 'it's no big deal.'
- Ignore the abusive behavior.

*   *   *   *   *

My mother was what I used to call a "selective" non-violent mom. What I mean is that she didn't believe in violence to solve problems or protect yourself for that matter. Yet, on the other hand, she had no problem unleashing on me when she had to discipline me. I clearly remember as a child being troubled by the fact that, every time I told my mother about an incident in school, her first response was, "What did you do to cause the fight?"

Now granted, I was one to fight back especially after my brush with being bullied. However, coming home and sharing how I had to defend myself and not getting the support from my mother bothered me for years. It especially bothered me when I would go to my friends' homes and hear their parents supporting them by saying, "Don't let anybody put their hands on you. I'm going to the school tomorrow and address this."

*   *   *   *   *

It's important that you make time to have a conversation, but let your child do the talking. Your job is to ask carefully worded questions about the situation and not about what your child may or may not have done. It is also important that you not go into a fighting mentality with your child.

Don't encourage your child to get physically aggressive with a bully, and don't fly off the handle which may cause your child to worry about what you might do. If they are worried that you are going to confront the bully or make a big deal about the situation, they might not feel safe talking to you about these issues in the future. It is important to stay calm and even keeled with the situation.

When having a conversation with your child about bullying, give him the power by allowing him to think about solutions on how to deal with the bully such as ways to change the bullying behavior. When your child feels empowered and has possibilities of what can be done, your child will be more likely to stand-up to the bully. This can be a very effective step toward stopping abusive behavior.

It is also important that you figure out what your child needs to do to feel better about the situation. If he can find a solution, it can be very empowering. Yet, your child may want your help since he simply may not know what to do. It is okay to give them suggestions and to offer your help.

It is important to keep in touch with your child about any bullying that they are experiencing. If things don't improve, you do need to step in and try to help the situation. If things escalate and your child starts to feel physically threatened, you might have to get authorities involved.

Any time there are threats of violence, you need to take this seriously. Any threats of violence need to be reported to the police immediately.

*   *   *   *   *

While finalizing this book, one of my staff members shared with me how she had to go to her daughter's school to address the principal about her child being kicked and punched by three boys. When she arrived at the school, she spoke to the teacher, asking what was going to be done about the boys that attacked her child. The teacher's response was very nonchalant and made it seem like it wasn't a big deal. She then said that the boys would be suspended.

The next day, one of the boys hit her daughter on the bus and, when my staff member went to the office, she was told that the principal was busy and wouldn't be able to speak to her at the moment. She told them that she would wait until she's available. She sat right outside of the principal's office and waited. The principal finally walked out, and the admin staff that initially shunned her were now trying their best to appear accommodating.

Long story short, the teacher lied to her, stating that the boys were suspended the same day. Not only were the kids not suspended, but the parents were also not even made aware of the situation. My staff member was also told numerous times that she would receive a return phone call from the teacher and principal. She eventually had to get the police and school board involved to resolve this situation and ultimately protect her child.

*   *   *   *   *

Your child needs to feel secure, and they can't feel that way if they think someone is going to harm them.
Make sure your child knows that bullying is wrong, no matter what. Having your support and understanding is the most important thing that you can do to help your

child through this difficult time. Make sure they know how brave and courageous it is to talk about what is going on. Give them your assurance that you all are going to handle this problem together and that they have your full support.

The above covers many points of conversation that you can have with your child and the steps you can take with the school, but your child is going to need some steps that they can take right away. The most important thing is that they feel safe. By making a plan for what they can do in the meantime will help them to feel better about going back to school.

Here are some short-term solutions to helping your child deal with the bully while you work on longer term solutions to the problem:

- *Avoid Them.* If your child can avoid the bully, this is one of the simplest steps they can take. If they know where the bully typically hangs out at school, it should be easy for them to stay out of their way.

- *Walk Away.* When confronted by the bully, don't stand there and take it. Walk away.

- *Tell Them to Stop.* If your child is confronted by a bully, tell them to stop their behavior and then act completely uninterested in what they are doing. This is another good time to walk away.

- *Find an Adult.* If they know that the bully is going to try and corner them, they should report that to an adult as quickly as possible.

- *Take Away Temptation.* If your child knows that the bully is going to try and take their money, have them leave their wallet at home. Don't let them bring the items that the bully is going to try and take away from them.

- *Buddy Up.* If there are times or areas of the school where the bully is unavoidable, see if you can get a friend to go with you. Bullies are less likely to attack when there is more than one person.

These are solutions to deal with non-violent bully attacks. If the situation escalates to physical abuse, your child must be prepared to defend himself or herself.

Getting your child involved with activities where the bully isn't located is a great way to give their self-confidence a strong boost. This will open them up to new experiences and get them away from the daily routine of the bully. Plus, this opens the opportunity for them to make new friends and do something different.

NEGATIVE PEER PRESSURE
Peer pressure can be a big part of bullying. It has long been proven that children are highly influenced by their friends. Having a higher status in peer groups is a big reason for being influenced to do things that the same child might not do on their own.

Children who are in peer groups that are considered popular are more likely to bully and participate in aggression towards other kids. Most often this is the indirect form of bullying that can go unnoticed by school authorities.

Peer pressure is more likely to garner bullying in the form of gossip, rumors, and rejection. The kids that are considered popular will encourage other children to behave this way. If you are concerned that your child might be making some wrong choices when it comes to their friendships, there are things you can do to get them on a better track.

What is important is to start conversations with your kids when they are young. The younger you start to bring up these important issues, the better. Developing kind and caring kids starts when they are young, if you wait until they get into school, it might just be too late.

Here are a few conversational tactics to help you set up good friendship boundaries with your kids:

- **What Makes a Good Friend?** – By asking your kids this question, you will open up a dialogue that helps them start to paint a picture of who would be a good friend and who wouldn't.

- **What is Bullying Behavior?** – With this question, you can help your kids see when bullying behavior is happening around them. Most kids don't want to be viewed as a bully by their peers. When you can narrow down what bullying behavior looks like, they will be able to make better choices.

- **Create Self-Esteem in Your Child** – When people believe in their own self-worth, they are less likely to be bullied or allow bullying behavior to happen around them. Get your kids involved in activities that foster good self-esteem. Studies show that this will not only help them not get bullied, but it can also help with other areas of peer pressure.

- *Meet Your Child's Friends* – If your child has a close friend at school, invite that child over to your house to play or spend the night. This can give you first-hand experience of what that friend is like and a clue of what is going on with your own child while at school. If you can drive your kids and their friends to an event, take it. While in the car, kids tend to talk more freely, thinking that you are not paying attention. This is an easy way to hear what really might be going on with them.

CHAPTER 14
BULLY PREVENTION PROGRAMS

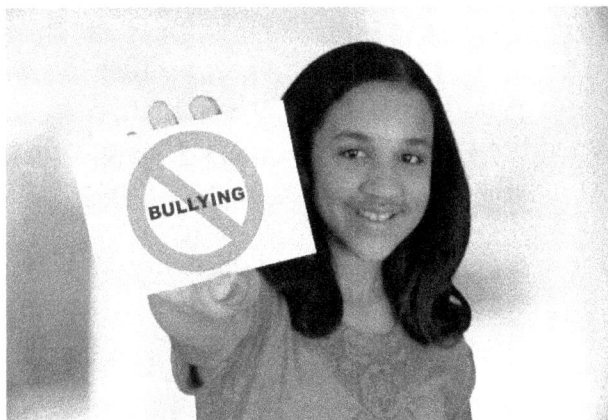

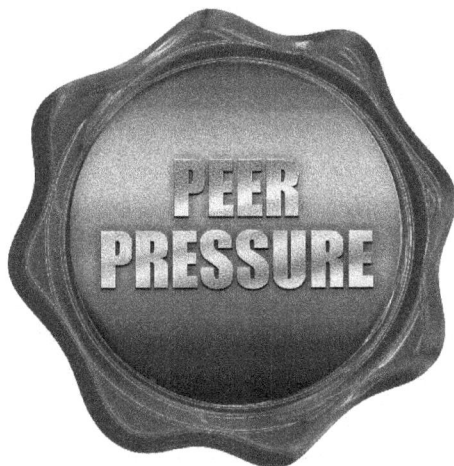

Many organizations work to stop bullying in schools. Many of these groups will come to school at no charge to help train parents, teachers, administrators, and students on what to do about bullying.

It seems that bully prevention works. Most bully prevention programs work to empower the target of bullying to stand up to their aggressors. They also work to help parents and teacher report bullying behavior and show bystanders what they can do to help stop bullying when they see it. All this work goes towards creating a school atmosphere where bullying is not tolerated.

These programs will also work closely with parents whose children have been known to cause issues around bullying other students. These programs can help parents alleviate aggression at home. This can work to stop parental aggression from being taken out on the child, which is often where kids first learn the behavior of bullying.

Bully prevention programs are educational tools to help explain what bullying really is and how to stop it from happening.

The programs work to teach kids that everyone has to work together to prevent bullying from happening. It shows the harmful effects that bullying can have on both the target and the bully and it helps give samples of other ways to communicate and interact that aren't abusive.

- ## BYSTANDERS AND WITNESSES

Often, training programs begin with identifying bystanders or witnesses. Children might not realize that, as a witness, they are a part of the bullying. The first step in bully prevention is to identify what it means to be a witness and what a witness should do if they see bullying happening around them.

One simple way to do this is to set up a scenario before starting the class. This could be something as simple as having another teacher walk in, set something on the desk and walk out. Or you could throw a paper airplane across the room.

By doing something unexpected, you will get them interested in what is going to happen. With kids, it is important that you don't just lecture. They have a shorter attention span, so anytime you talk for longer than ten minutes you will have lost them. Instead, break-up what you say with interactive activities and conversations where you just ask questions, and they come up with the solutions.

Once you have started the training by doing something unexpected, start to ask them questions to engage them in conversation. Start with questions like:

Who saw what just happened?
Have the kids raise their hands for those who did witness the activity. When you have a good idea of the number of kids who witnessed the action, move on to the next question.

Who was aware something happened, but didn't know what it was?

Again, have the kids raise their hands and see who might have noticed that something happened or knew something had happened but didn't know what it was.

Who can describe exactly what took place?
For this question, call on one or two students to explain exactly what happened. Let them use as much detail as they can. Your job is to just listen at this point. Don't try and lead them to answer specifically or steer their answer towards one course. Just let them be open to what they want to say.

At this point, you explain that all the people in the classroom that knew what happened were witnesses to the event. When talking about bullying, the same explanation applies. Those who know what is going on, whether they saw it, heard it, or just knew something had happened are witnesses. And being a witness to bullying is essential to stopping bullying.

From this point in your bullying prevention training, you move into a more conversational tone. Again, you are going to ask them questions, but leave more space for them to answer by telling a story or giving as much, or as little, detail as they want to.

Ask the children the following questions:
- Have you ever witnessed a bullying situation?
- How did you feel about it?

Now you will explain to them that, anyone who actually sees a bullying scenario take place is called a bystander. These are people who not only know that something happened, but actually watched it happen.

From there you move into interactive presentations. Use a projector or large pictures to show scenes of bullying taking place. Tell a story about what is happening in the scene and get the children to answer questions about who is the bully, who is the target, who is the bystander, and who is the witness.

Once the kids start to understand the different roles in a bullying scenario, they will begin to have a better understanding of what can be done when bullying is happening in front of them. They will begin to see that the bystander and witnesses are just as involved as the bully and the target.

During this process, it is important to check in with the kids and ask them about their feelings and what they think the feelings of the children in the scene might be. When they can connect their own feelings to those of the kids in the scene, they will have a better grasp of how bullying can feel, even if they have never experienced it on their own.

Once you have created this understanding, ask them the following questions:

- How could a bystander be a part of the problem?
- If you were being bullied and there were bystanders around you, how would you feel?
- What might the bully be thinking about the bystanders?
- How could the bystanders be a part of the solution to stop the bullying?

From this point, you can start to talk about the solutions that can help the bullying situation from the bystander's perspective. Ask the students what the bystanders could do to change what is happening. Start a conversation about actions that can be taken that will help the bullying to stop, while keeping everyone safe.

At this point, you might need to stop and take a break or end the training. Remember, kids can only take in so much information before they start to feel overloaded. Bully prevention training should happen over a longer period of time and not be crammed all into one day.

By spreading it out over a few weeks, you also give the children time to integrate what they have learned. Often times there will be incidents that come up during the space of the trainings where they get to use the skills that you are teaching them.

When you come back to the training, it is good to start off by asking the students if they saw any bullying since the last gathering. And if so, what could they have done about it. Be careful here. This could lead to tattle-telling or finger-pointing. With younger kids, this might not be an area you want to tread on, but with older kids, they are usually more diplomatic with sharing.

• RESPECT

In your next session, find a story that outlines a bullying scenario. There are many books, stories, and training materials that are explicitly geared towards bully preventions trainings. Once you read the story to the class, open the floor for conversation again.

Do this by asking questions.

Ask them how they think the characters were feeling. It is also a good idea to ask what they would have done if they were in each of the character's positions.

"What would you do if you were the bystander in this story?"
You can also ask the kids what advice they would offer to the characters or what the characters could have done differently to have a better outcome.

From this point, it is a good idea to introduce the concept of respect. Once upon a time, most school age children understood the concepts of do unto others. That is no longer the case, and part of bully preventions programs is to teach this concept.

Ask the children if they know what respect means. As they give their answers, write some of the keywords on the board. Then give the actual definition of respect: *Respect means treating others as you would want to be treated.*

From there ask the kids to share times that they have been respectful or to share a story of what it means to have respect for another person. You can now split the kids into pairs and have them make lists of activities that they could do with a friend. From here you are making the connection of respect to friendship.

When children feel like they have a friendship with other kids they are less likely to engage in bullying behavior. This is why smaller classrooms and smaller schools have fewer instances of bullying. The kids feel a closer connection to each other, and they look at all of the other students as friends.

This builds better connections between the children and makes it in such a way they are less likely to bully or pick on each other.

When the groups are done, have them share their lists of what you can do to cultivate friendships. Encourage them to use these things during the break between your next class meeting. Let them know that you are going to be sharing their stories when you gather together again. This will help the kids to pay attention to opportunities where they can offer respectful behavior to each other between your sessions.

At your next session, have one or two of the kids tell their stories of how they were respectful to another person since your last training. Don't open this up for a lot of conversation. Just let it be a point where the kids can share their triumphs since you were last together. If it feels appropriate, have the group clap for the story and congratulate them on being respectful and developing friendships.

• PROBLEMS AND SOLUTIONS

To really make a difference in bullying, the kids need to understand that they are each powerful enough to offer solutions. Moving forward in the bullying prevention training you want to give the kids a problem and encourage them to help you discover a good solution.

This should be done as both an individual working process and a group process. It is good to start with the individual and then move into the group, but either way is fine. The following are questions that can be asked for either the individual process or the group process.

For the individual work, have the students write the questions on a piece of paper and then give them a limited amount of time to write their thoughts on the questions. Once that time is up, have two or three of the kids share what they have written.

For the group process, break the kids up into groups of three or four individuals. Have them discuss the questions and write down their thoughts or potential solutions. Have a card written up that you give to each of the groups with the following instructions:

- Allot time for each person to share their thoughts and ideas.
- Listen when others are speaking.
- Stay on the subject.
- Be respectful to each other.

Here are the questions that can be used for this section. Remember, they can be used for either the solitary writing portion or for the group discussion.

- Explain how people can be part of the bullying problem, even if they are not the bully.

- What would happen if no one reported the instances of bullying?

- Why is it so important that everyone take responsibility to stop bullying?

- Should older students help younger students to stop bullying?

- What are specific things that will help to stop bullying?

- What does it mean to be a bystander and what should a bystander do when they see bullying happen? Upon completion of this segment, be sure to encourage them with lots of praise as they break and prepare for their next session.

Next, as you move forward, you will start to explore what it means to bully.

• WHAT IS BULLYING?

When you gather back again, it is good to open conversation and see where the kids might have been able to use their skills to stop negative events from taking place. You will be surprised where kids will see areas of disrespect and how brave they are to speak up when they know it is okay to do so.

In this area of the bully prevention training, you want to start to explore what bullying really means. This is another good place to break into groups and talk about bullying behavior.

Kids might not realize all the ways that someone can be bullying others. Often in these breakout sessions, you will learn that many kids think of bullying as being physically aggressive or teasing someone, but they don't often think about exclusion as a means of bullying.

Purposely leaving children out of games and activities is a form of bullying. Introducing this concept to kids is important, and it will build off of the lessons on respect that you have already introduced.

When the kids are finished exploring what bullying actually is in their groups, have each group share what they came up with. Make sure that you build on the topics that they introduce and include any areas where they might have missed.

Depending on the age of the children you are working with, this can be a great place to introduce role-playing games to work with bullying. Choose several volunteers to enact scenes where different types of bullying are taking place. Let the kids in the class pause the scene to point out where there is an opportunity to do something different and change the direction of the bullying from happening.

It is important through this process that the kids come to understand that bullying is not about avoiding disagreements. Disagreements are normal, and as long as people remain cool and calm, they are a good way to get to understand each other's point of view. Bullying is something altogether different.

Bullying is done to cause harm to the other person. This could be physical or emotional harm. Bullying is an entirely one-sided activity with the bully being the only one that gains anything. It can leave the target feeling isolated and hurt.

Developing a common language for the kids is going to go a long way in bully prevention. Occasionally bullying happens because the children don't understand that there are being insensitive to other people. They are learning social skills at school along with math and reading. Helping them to develop strong and healthy social skills is important. With a common language, the kids are going to be less likely to bully and will stand up to bullying when it does happen.

This process alone can take up an entire meeting session. Again, it is important not to give too much information. Introduce one basic concept at each meeting time and allot time for the children to be a part of the discussion. It is also good to space out the session so that the kids can implement some of the lessons that you all have been working on together.

- ### STOPPING BULLYING

Once you create the common language and the kids understand what behaviors are considered bullying, you can teach them how to stop bullying when it happens. This is a two-pronged approach to bully prevention.

First, you want to teach them how to stop a bully when they are on the receiving end of the abuse. Second, you want to teach them how to stop a bully when they are a bystander.

Some of this you would have already created a framework for in your previous sessions of class time.

The first part of stopping a bully is to teach the kids to stand up for themselves. When a child understands that they have a right not to be teased, pushed around, or bullied, they are more likely to do this anyway, but there are good ways to approach this to help them develop higher communication skills.

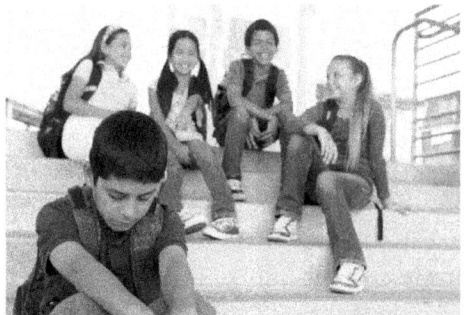

To start this process, have the kids share ways to stop a bully and write these things on the board. Once you have a list of several items, go through each of them and discuss. It is likely that the kids will suggest ways to stop bullying that are not the appropriate way to respond. It will be up to you as the facilitator to turn that around and show them a better way to deal with that situation.

Here are a few dos and don'ts for you to be ready for when you have this conversation with the kids:

- **No Fighting** – If someone suggests fighting back, you want to turn this around. Remember, this is about respect. If you are showing someone respect, even a bully, you would not want to fight with them. Instead, encourage them to use their words and find another way that does not include being physical. Remember that fighting often makes things worse and can lead to more problems down the road.

- **Getting Help** – If the kids suggest telling a teacher or a parent, this should be highly encouraged. Help the kids to understand that a teacher isn't going to be mad, but rather the teacher is going to help them find a better way to communicate with each other and stop the bullying from happening.

- **Finding a Buddy** – This may or may not come up, but it is good to explain to kids that a bully is less likely to pick on you if you are with a group of friends. If they are worried about being bullied, encourage them to ask a friend to hang out with them or walk home with them to help stop bullying behavior from happening.

- **Tell Them to Stop** – Often you can stop a bully by telling them just that, to stop. When the bully knows that they are not going to get a reaction from you, it can often stop their behavior. Encourage the kids to breathe, stay calm, and tell the bully to stop. If this doesn't work, encourage them to walk away and find help.

Because you are creating a common language through this training, the kids are going to be less likely to bully each other in the first place. And, as they move through life and potentially experience bullying in other places, they will know how to deal with it constructively.

By doing the above steps, the kids will be standing up to bullies and potentially changing their behavior going forward. This can be difficult for kids who are not typically assertive. This is why it is important to give several options on what to do because not all kids are going to be willing to speak up or put themselves in a situation where they feel on the spot.

It is important to note that these kids are often the ones who get picked on the most, to begin with. When bullies think they have an easy mark, they are more likely to continue the abusive behavior.

- ### THE AGREEMENT

The final step in the bully prevention program is to have the students sign a pledge. This is an important part of the process and should be something that each of the kids feels honored and excited to do. They should have bought into the process at this point, so making this pledge and agreement should feel like the obvious thing to do.

You can either have a pre-written pledge that the students agree to or come up with the pledge together. Creating a pledge as a group can be a very powerful process and will ensure that the kids are more invested in the process, but it can also take a lot more time to develop.

One simple way to do both is to create a shell or outline for the pledge. Break the kids up into smaller groups and have them fill in the areas of the pledge together with their group. Each group then reports back what they have created by writing it on the board.

From here you will take the areas where all of the groups have written the same, or similar, ideas and use those to craft the pledge together.

Once you have it clearly written out, you then get the approval from the class by asking for a "thumbs up" sign from everyone who likes the pledge that you all have created together. At that point you have each of the students write the pledge out on a piece of paper and sign and date it. If you are using a pre-written pledge, follow this same process.

The pledge should touch on the following points:

- I will not bully others.

- I will not allow myself to be bullied.

- I will have respect for others.

- I will have respect for myself.

- If I see bullying happening, I will take steps to stop it.

Write the pledge on a large poster and hang it in the classroom as a constant reminder to the kids of the pledge that they have made around bullying and bully prevention.

Another final step that can be very powerful is to have the kids write a letter to their future selves about why respect is important and how they can stop bullying. Have them write this letter and put it in an envelope addressed to their home address. At the end of the school year mail all the letters.

This can be a powerful reminder to the kids about self-respect, respecting others, and stopping the abuse of bullying in their lives.

• WHY BULLY PREVENTION?

Typically, bully prevention should be started with kids at an early age, but this is an area that is relatively new to schools. Starting in the 2nd or 3rd grade is the most powerful time. If you start there, it is good to have a refresher or follow up class in the remaining grade, through high school.

If bully prevention is a newer idea to your school, starting in 4th, 5th, or 6th grade can also work and be very impactful for the kids who go through the training.

The bully prevention tends to do a lot more than just stop bullying behaviors at schools. It can also help kids to have high self-esteem and feel secure in pointing out other areas in their lives where they feel they are not being respected. This can help them to do better in school, create strong friendships, and develop positive attitudes around relationships and interactions.

Some of the coping skills that children will learn through bully prevention are as follows:

- *Assertiveness:* When a child stands up for themselves, this is the most powerful thing they can do to stop being bullied. Too often kids don't even realize that they are allowed to stand up for themselves and tell the bully to stop. Teaching children how to be assertive and say what they need will lead to them having better interpersonal skills.

- Research also shows that the way the target handles the initial bullying will determine the result of the bullying as well as if it continues to happen over time or not. If children are aggressive in response to the bullying, it is more likely that it will continue to happen. If children ignore the problem or get emotionally rattled the bullying is also likely to continue. But if children are assertive and speak up against the behaviors, the bullying behavior is less likely to continue.

- *Emotional Control:* It is not unusual to get emotional when being abused and it isn't always easy to stop yourself from feeling emotional when being bullied. One of the ways that bully prevention helps to stop bullying is by teaching kids how to control their emotions and not let them get carried away with anger, aggression, or sadness when confronted with a bully. When a target can calmly tell the bully to stop their behavior, it works the majority of the time.

- *Social Skills:* Working through a bully prevention system teaches kids how to work together and be successful in building relationships. This will help them far into their adult lives, in their work, and in their relationships. Not to mention that children with many friends tend to have fewer issues with being bullied in the first place and have less long-term harmful effects when they are bullied.

- *Shared Beliefs:* Since a group of students go through the bully prevention trainings together, they grow up with a shared set of beliefs. This will encourage them to take what they have learned out into the world beyond their classroom. This can help to stop bullying in other places, like after-school activities, where the other children might not have been through the same training system.

Not only is bully prevention training important for the students, but these programs can also help parents and teachers to see what works and what doesn't when it comes to changing abusive behavior. When everyone, including staff and families are speaking the same language around bullying, the message goes much deeper into the children.

- **TEACHER BUY-IN**

Too often teachers don't understand the full effects that bullying can have on their students. Many still regard bullying as typical childhood antics and don't take the necessary steps to stop it from happening or prevent it.

In fact, a recent study revealed that up to 25 percent of teachers don't feel it necessary to intervene when they see bullying happening to their students.

Studies show that when teachers are connected to training for bully prevention, they are more likely to succeed. Too often teachers don't even realize that bullying is happening. This is because the children are smart enough to do it out of their sights.

But when teachers and school staff go through training about recognizing bullying behaviors and the target's reactionary behaviors, it can help to stop bullying much faster.
Training teachers on bullying also helps them to feel more empowered. Teachers don't receive training on how to deal with bullies or what to do with children who get bullied.

When they do see something happening, they often don't have the skills to handle the situation.

By training the teachers on bully prevention, they will receive the tools that they need to help their students better. It helps to improve their skills in recognizing that bullying is occurring, stepping in effectively, and having the skills to stopping it before it gets out of control. These steps not only help the students to feel more secure and know that their teachers are supporting them, but it also helps the teachers to have a better grasp of their classrooms and students.

It is important that teachers are on board when it comes to bullying prevention. Teachers need to understand that when they don't intervene with bullying, they are allowing it to happen. This makes them just as guilty of the behavior as the bully. When the victims don't feel supported or safe with the adults at their school, they are more likely to withdraw, not report abuse, and suffer emotionally.

This can lead to kids falling behind in class and being out sick from school more often. These behaviors of avoidance only cause them to fall further behind in their classes, which can lead to more bullying. All of this can be avoided when teachers are paying attention and help to stop bullying in their classrooms.

Chapter 15
How Schools Can Make a Difference

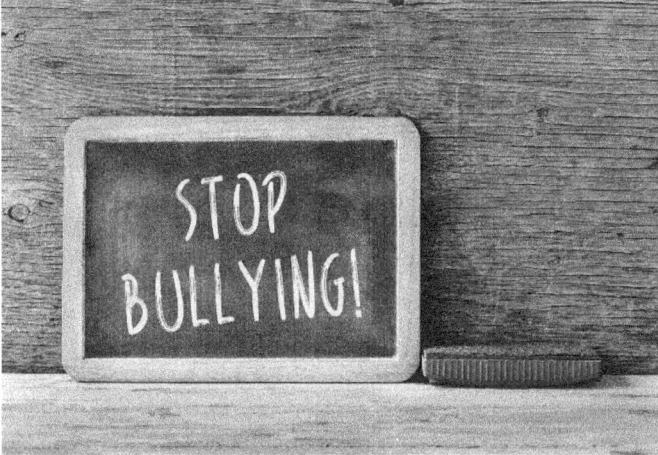

CREATING A BULLY-FREE SCHOOL

There are many ways that schools can change bullying from the inside out. Creating a bully prevention program at your school is not as difficult as you might think. Some schools opt to pay for outside training resources to help them implement trainings and bully prevention in their schools, but it doesn't have to be that complicated, and it doesn't have to cost any money.

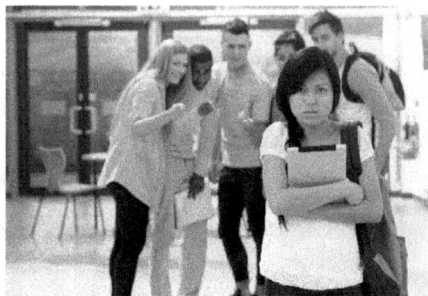

What it does require is a dedication from the school, the administration, the teachers, and the parents of the students to learn new ways of operating and changing the culture of bullying on their campuses.

Here are some ways to change your school culture to one that embraces a no bullying policy:

- **Assess** – Before you go down the road of training and creating a culture of a bully-free zone, it is essential to determine what is happening in your school around bullying already. The best way to do this is to send out an anonymous survey to the staff and students about the bullying they have witnessed and experienced.

- **Create a Team** – Find a group of people, teachers, and parents that are ready to spearhead the bully free policies that you want to implement. It is good to have a wide array of people who want to work on the project. It is also good to keep your team smaller, four to five people; otherwise, it will be hard to get things accomplished.

- **Involvement** – You want to get teachers, staff, and students involved with the project. You might come up against some resistance because there will be teachers who don't feel that this is necessary. There will be staff members who think they don't need to go through training, but don't let these things stop you from making a difference in your school's policies.

- **Code of Conduct** – Whether you enlist a training program right away or not, you want to develop a code of conduct for the students and staff. This should be a form that outlines what behavior is unacceptable and gives personal responsibility to each of the students and teachers to behave in a healthy, respectful manner. Each student should sign this code of conduct and have their parents sign it too. You should have each teacher sign this code of conduct, and the code should be posted around campus as a reminder.

- **Create Bullying Consequences** – If your students don't know what the consequences are for bullying behavior, they are more likely to act out in ways that bully others. Make it clear what the implications are for bullying other students. This shouldn't just be punishment, but rather trainings and teachings that help these students to stop their abusive behavior.

- **Make a Safe Space for Reporting** – Too often students don't report when they have been bullied because of a fear of repercussions. Children are also told from a very early age not to be a "tattle-tale." This can be a confusing message for kids. Students need to understand that bullying is abuse, and they should not put up with it. They should be encouraged to come forward when they are bullied or when they see others being bullied. You can also offer an anonymous system for reporting where students can write their experience and put it into a locked box where they won't be singled out for reporting.

- **Make Supervision a Priority** – In order to ensure that bullying isn't happening at your school, you need to make sure that students are being supervised all the time. School staff should have a handle on what is happening with students both on and off the campus – before and after school.

- **Teach Skills** – Using bully prevention training is going to make students to start developing the skills that will stop bullying, but this is something that needs to be an ongoing process at your school. One training isn't going to change everything forever.

- Implement ongoing trainings to help kids continue to develop the social skills they need to stop bullying when they see it.

- **Integrate** – Don't just set aside time to do bully prevention training and always have it labeled as such. What is important is for your teachers to integrate these lessons into their regular lesson plans. By reinforcing what the kids learned in their bully prevention into other unrelated school activities, the kids will absorb the information more easily.

- **Parent Involvement** – It has been proven time and time again that parents who are involved with their children's education have kids that do better in school. Getting parents involved with bully prevention can be as easy as having parent night meetings once a month where you talk about these issues. If that seems unlikely, you can send home memos with the kids or have the teachers talk about the bully prevention programs during parent-teacher conferences.

- Working with parents can be difficult. This is especially true if their child has been accused of bullying. You have to help teach parents better ways to deal with their children, although this can be tricky to navigate. Not all parents are going to be willing to hear what you have to say. Remember: bullies are often repeating behavior that they've seen in their homes.

- **Create Protocol** – Once you have the consequences outlined, you need to create a protocol for when someone is accused of or caught bullying another student. It is important to talk separately to all the children involved. It is also good to monitor the child that has been accused more closely and to make sure that the parents get involved. There could be underlying reasons for the child acting out. You might need to do more investigating to what is going on than what appears to be happening on the surface.

- **Reinforce the Positive** – Punishments don't work. What works is to reinforce the positive behavior. When you reward a student for making positive changes or doing the right thing, you are more likely to see more of the behavior that you want. It is also important to give the victim tools to deal with the bully and help to boost their self-confidence in case something happens again.

- **Off-Campus Bullying** – One of the problems with bullying is that it often happens outside the school campus. This is one of the reasons that it usually goes unnoticed by school staff and teachers. It is important that you reinforce the code of conduct that you have created to apply to the students when they are off campus as well as on campus. This code of conduct should be implemented anytime they are dealing with another student. Including walking home, on the bus, off-campus school events, on the internet, and anytime they see each other in public. It is harder to enforce this behavior off of school grounds, but it is vital that the students understand that this is expected of them.

CHAPTER 16
MYTHS ABOUT BULLIES AND VICTIMS

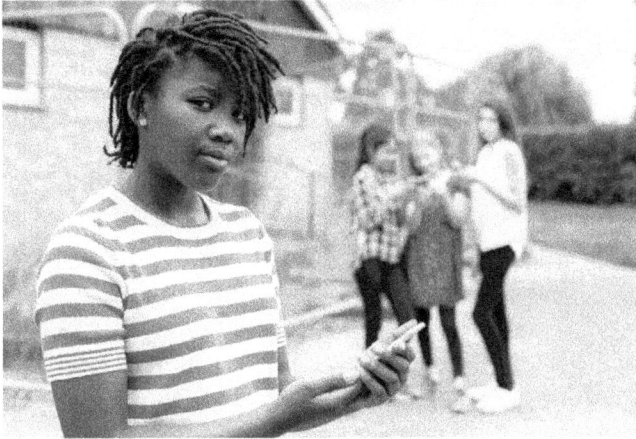

There is a lot of false information out there about bullies and the children that they target. Too often kids are told to ignore the bully and they will go away, but this is proving to be bad advice. It was once thought that bullies suffered from low self-esteem, but this isn't exactly accurate either. So, what is the truth about bullies and the victims of their behavior?

Here are a few myths about bullies and what the truth really is:

- **Myth: Bullies have low self-esteem.**
- *Fact:* It is now understood that most bullies have an inflated sense of self. These people tend to think that they are better than other people. They don't have low self-esteem, but their sense of self is skewed so that they can't see the reality of who they are. They choose to pick on others to help them continue to feel superior to others.

- **Myth: Bullies have no friends.**
- *Fact:* Bullies actually tend to be very popular and have many friends. This ability to dominate others helps them to bring people towards them and have large social circles. Sometimes bullying happens as a way for these people to hold on to their high social status by not letting others get ahead of them on the social ladder.

- **Myth: Bullying only affects the bully and the victim.**
- *Fact:* Studies show that the children who witness bullying develop just as many social anxiety issues as the children who are the victims of the attacks. Bullying often happens with witnesses and these

kids will often suffer as well or edge the bully on and become bullies themselves.

- **Myth: Being a victim makes you stronger.**
- *Fact:* This isn't always the case. Some people can overcome being the victim of bullying and go on to have normal lives, but many people also suffer emotional scarring that lasts their entire lives. The severity of the bullying can cause serious psychological implications.

- **Myth: There is a victim personality.**
- *Fact:* This has yet to be proven. In many cases, it is unclear if the victim started out on the outside of the social circle or was pushed outside of the social circle. What is true is that children who don't stand up for themselves when they are bullied are more likely to be bullied again.

- **Myth: Victims of bullying are more likely to be violent.**
- *Fact:* The opposite is actually true. Children who are bullied are more likely to suffer alone than to fight back violently. Obviously, there have been cases where children have fought back violently, but this is rare. A victim is more likely to commit suicide than murder. Studies do show that bullies are more likely to engage in violent crimes as they age.

- **Myth: Bullies are not victims and vice versa.**
- *Fact:* Bullies are just as likely to be victims of another bully, and often victims will turn around and bully others. There is no clear avenue between who is a bully and who is a victim.

- **Myth: Bullies are easy to spot.**
- *Fact:* Bullies tend to be highly manipulative. Often you will have no idea who the bully is in the classroom. They are not only good at picking on the other kids and not getting caught, but they are good at getting the adults to believe them.

- **Myth: Bullying will always have some form of physicality.**
- *Fact:* Physical bullying is a reality, but the emotional and mental bullying is much more likely to happen. When a child is beaten up, it is a lot harder to hide than if they are teased mercilessly. Children are more likely to be abused and bullied in other ways rather than physically.

- **Myth: A bully will be the biggest kid.**
- *Fact:* Physical size has nothing to do with whether someone will be a bully or not. It is more about not being able to handle their aggression than their size. Plus, not all bullying is about being able to dominate another person physically. Many times, bullies will be passive aggressive, use manipulation, coercion, or other underhanded means to control the victim.

- **Myth: Boys are more likely to be bullied than girls.**
Fact: Girls are more likely to be bullied. A 2007 survey revealed that 34 percent of girls had felt bullied at one time, while only 31 percent of boys reported the same thing.

CHAPTER 17
BUILDING SELF-ESTEEM THROUGH MARTIAL ARTS

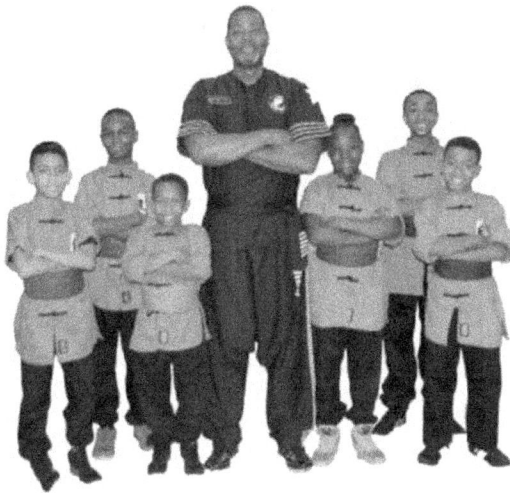

Self-esteem is the antidote to bullying as well as the vaccine. A confident child can put off bullies with both their speech and behavior. Confidence is a difficult thing to inspire in a child. We used to think that confidence could be instilled by simply telling children that they were exceptional. We created the concept of participation trophies and ribbons in order to boost self-esteem.

We eliminated sports that made children feel inferior. We stopped grading in red ink to avoid hurting feelings. Unfortunately, it was all for naught. Ill-gotten self-esteem that results from unearned accolades is a fleeting thing. Children require more than empty words in order to trust that they are capable. Children excel and feel exceptional when their parents set them up for success.

Studies continue to show that the most resilient and confident children are those whose parents have enrolled them in some sort of extracurricular skill or sport. Put simply, the best thing you can do for your child's self-esteem is put them in a position to train at a skill. Training allows them to build confidence in their ability to take action and make changes in the world around them. Physical training, in particular, gives them a feel for how their body functions in the world and how physically capable they can truly be.

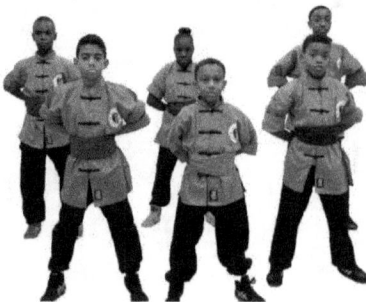

Enrolling your children in a martial arts class will allow them to build confidence as they build competence.

Unlike their peers, your child will have a real and actionable skill which they can demonstrate to others. This will give them the confidence required to stand up to a bullying attack, without them ever throwing a punch. Not only will the process of studying a martial art build your child's confidence, but it will also prepare them to stand up for themselves and others. Martial arts emphasize the importance of protecting those you care for. Kids who study martial arts are unlikely to be bystanders. Instead, they are the kind of students who take action in order to protect not only themselves, but those around them.

*   *   *   *   *

At my school, one of the procedures we've implemented when one of our students is being bullied is a simple school visitation with six to eight of my Blackbelt students. It works like this: once the parent notifies the school that their child is going to be visited by his/her martial arts instructor, we show-up and sit with the child in class and during lunch. We simply sit and laugh with our student and the student's friends as an example of how we should treat one another.

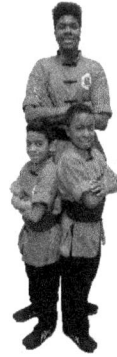

Those simple steps have worked miracles because we never had to address anyone. At times, we gave quick talks with the kids about bullying and answered their questions about martial arts. Our parents feel good knowing that they have a place to turn to for help when things get out of hand.

*   *   *   *   *

THE IMPORTANCE OF MENTORSHIP

One of the most tragic symptoms of our modern era is the reduction in connections between not only peers, but people of different age groups. With this increasing isolation, we have created entire generations of young people who have no experience with the concept of mentorship. Mentorship serves an essential component in the lives of children. Through careful guidance from trusted adults, children develop a nuanced understanding of what it is to be an upstanding member of the society. They receive additional input about the difference between right and wrong as well as advice about how to handle various aspects of their lives.

A child's relationship with their mentors provides their parents with an objective view into their successes and struggles. A child's mentor can provide you with valuable information:

- Who your child associates with,
- What your child does, and
- Your child's challenges.

Martial arts emphasize the mentorship between an instructor and those receiving instruction. Children are encouraged to ask questions and discuss how they've used their training. Discussions with their martial arts instructor can help children work through bullying and find positive solutions to the issues that they face.

Imagine this situation:

A nine-year-old child walks through the halls of his middle school and another student, one or two grades higher than him, sees an opportunity to take advantage of someone smaller than him. He walks up to him and pushes him against the wall and makes a quiet threat in order to erase any chance of retaliation. The nine-year-old has no experience in this situation, so doesn't know what to do and in his mind cannot go to anyone.

Sometime later, the same bully approaches the child during a meeting in an auditorium. There are witnesses everywhere, teachers at the bottom of the stage and students in the stands. The bully sits right next to the child and issues another threat. This encounter is a bit different, however. At the end of the issued threat, the bully slaps our nine-year-old, sending his head bouncing off the concrete wall. He is left in tears and feels ashamed.

Remember, there are other students next to him and teachers at the stage, but the bully isn't so much as looked at by anyone. Call it fear, probable denial or whatever you want, things have escalated, and the danger is far higher now. It's a new school year, and the bully has moved to high school, and our nine-year-old is now 10 or 11 and in his last year of junior high. This time, however, some punk kid looks at him wrongly and he doesn't like it. He goes to the student of a lower grade than he and shoves him a little, making sure that he knows who's boss. For good measure, he issues a threat so that he has no fear of retaliation later.

This is a tragic story that happens over and over again in schools all across America. There are many times the situation could have been dealt with in a nonviolent and acceptable manner. There could have been hall monitors to stop the first incident; there could have been teachers supervising students in the auditorium instead of trying to play hero with the failing electronic systems, or there could have been a student elected body the student could have gone to and feel safe talking to other peers. None of this occurred.

Let's replay the situation out a couple of different ways now: In the first instance, let's say that before encountering the bully, our initial nine-year-old had martial arts training. This training gave him the confidence to stand up to the bully and be upfront about his intentions. He'd have the confidence to issue his own ultimatum of reporting the bully to the nearest authority or warn the bully that, if he touched him, he would sustain bodily harm.

In this instance, the bully would most certainly back off, and the situation would have been over before it had a chance to begin. The teachers would have been involved immediately, and an investigation would ensue about the home life of said bully fixing the problem where it lives. If attacked, the nine-year-old could have successfully defended himself (as he has every right in American to do so) and not feel overwhelming fear and shame in the wake of an unscrupulous bully.

In the second instance, let's say that after the first instance of violence, our nine-year-old had friends who took martial arts classes. He asks them about those classes, and they invite him one night, and he promptly begins classes with the permission of his parents. In one fell swoop, our nine-year-old has put himself into a group of other like-minded and strong peers. Strength in numbers. He is learning ethical ways to deal with would be bullies. He is gaining confidence in himself and his peers. The next time the said bully comes calling, he doesn't need to "beat them up," his peers are there to back him. Now he has witnesses to the attempt, and the proper authorities can be notified by a number of students instead of one. Squeaky wheels get the grease. In either case, bullying would have been thwarted because like most predators, they seek the weakest of the group, the one most likely not to hit them back.

The best way to deal with bullying is to prevent it from the start. In our story, the cycle of violence never ends. It happens to one, and the virus is contracted by another and then another and then another until you have a self-fulfilling prophecy that could end with an even more tragic story like a school shooting, suicide, or rape. The martial arts offer a simple solution that is both gratifying to the practitioners and is accessible to everyone at every age at every health level. Think about how much a child's life could change by practicing martial arts?

Martial arts take years of dedication to master and requires extreme focus to do well. If done so, the benefits last a literal lifetime and can be passed on from generation to generation.

Years ago, an experiment was commissioned to study the long-term effects of delaying instant gratification. Children were escorted into a room one at a time, and a marshmallow was put in front of them. They were given two choices, they could eat the marshmallow now and receive none in the future or they could wait a predetermined amount of time and receive multiple marshmallows later.

What the experiment found was that children who indulged in their instant gratification now experience less overall success later on in life. Less success in relationships, less success in both secondary and post-secondary school, and less success in their chosen careers fields. Children who delayed their need for instant gratification were shown to be much more successful later in life.

Delayed gratification tends to bring about more success in relationships, more success in both secondary and post-secondary school, and more success in their chosen careers fields. This proves that, if children undertake a skill that takes years of focus and dedication to complete, they are more likely to succeed in all areas of life long after they have left home. What could be a better gift to your child than a gift that they can rely on for years and years? Now imagine what a child could accomplish in their life as a result of practicing martial arts based on everything you've read so far. How much better of an existence would he or she experience as a result of one single decision? The decision to enroll a child into a long-term martial arts program will benefit a child for years to come.

CHAPTER 18
ACTION STEPS FOR ENROLLING YOUR CHILD INTO MARTIAL ARTS CLASSES

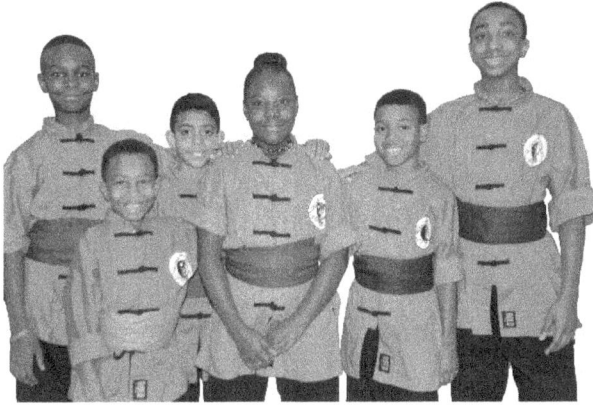

- Ask your child if any of their friends are taking classes.
- Google your local area for classes.
- Be sure your child is allowed to audit the class and several other classes first.
- Do a price comparison to weigh value and costs. If no such class exists in your area take these steps.

- At the next PTA meeting, mention a long-term meetup that you are setting up for martial arts classes for the kids.

- Gauge the level of interest of the group.
- Next, find private martial arts masters/teachers either in the surrounding area or on the internet.

- Their compensation will have to be worth their travel and time. So, at the next PTA meeting, discuss this with everyone.

QUESTIONS TO ASK THE MARTIAL ARTS SCHOOL OWNER

- How long have you been involved in the martial arts?
- What is the main focus of your program? (The answer should be to 'develop confident young leaders.')
- Do you have an anti-bullying program?
- Can you give me examples of incidents you had to address and what were the outcomes?

BONUS SECTION

- ➤ ADULT BULLYING
- ➤ THE BULLY BASICS – A QUICK REFERENCE GUIDE
- ➤ MORE BULLY TRAGEDIES – REAL LIFE STORIES

ADULT BULLYING (OR WORKPLACE BULLYING)

Although this book is primarily about child bullying, I wanted to add this section about adult bullying to help drive home the point about the effects of bullying.

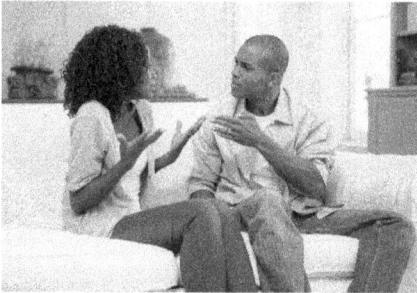

Children are not the only ones that experience bullying. In adults, bullying can happen in many different places, but the most common form of adult bullying is known as workplace bullying. Workplace bullying is actually very common and often seen as a way for higher ups, or management, to deal with subordinates.

The reality is that workplace bullying is considered a form of discrimination and can be viewed as dangerous and damaging workplace violence. Unfortunately, because it is used as a method of management, it is often very difficult to prove when bullying happens in the workplace.

Statistics show that one in six employees will experience bullying at work. Workplace bullying is more passive aggressive and less likely to turn into physical violence than the bullying that happens in childhood. Too often, people who bully in the office or workplace are within the code of conduct for their company. Since they are within what is allowed as far as the policies of the organization are concerned, their behavior often goes unreported and unpunished.

In many cases, especially with adults and in corporate environments, a bully mentality is tolerated. These environments can quickly become toxic, but no one feels that they have the power to stop the process. This behavior has been tolerated for years in the corporate world, with the revolving door of people who can no longer take the abuse clear to everyone except those who need to see it.

The best way to see if actual abuse and bullying is happening in an office or work environment is to look at the morale of the employees and the amount of turnover. Low morale and high turnover are often signs of workplace bullying, and such behavior is most likely coming from a member of management.

The difference between workplace bullying and management techniques is that the bully will focus on the person rather than the tasks assigned. Often this treatment can be rather vague, and people who are bullied may have a hard time explaining how the treatment is even abusive. Many employees are told to stop being so sensitive or to brush it off. Bullying should never be tolerated!

Don't be fooled into thinking that only certain personality types get bullied in the office. Practically anyone can end up with a bully for a boss or co-worker. This can happen to men and women of any race, religious, or sexual orientation. It can happen in both white collar and blue collar work environments and at any point in the chain of command.

Workplace bullying can look different than it does in children on the playground. In the workplace, people who experience bullying will often be purposely left out of meetings, put down in front of other employees, talked about behind their back, or forced to suffer different forms of humiliation. Any of these things could happen as an isolated incident, but over time a pattern of this treatment is a sign of bullying.

Here are some other specific signs that could indicate that you are being bullied at work:

- Being treated rudely by co-workers.
- Being yelled at.
- Not being invited to social events that are work-related.
- Employees arriving late only to meetings that you are heading.
- Being purposely ignored.
- Not being given praise for a job well done when deserved.
- Not receiving feedback on your job performance.
- Not being given help when requesting it.
- Being repeatedly put down about your competence.
- Having your communications ignored by others in the office.
- Having your work sabotaged.
- Being denied promotion without cause.
- Being the victim of mean pranks.
- Having a larger workload or shorter deadlines than other co-workers.
- Being accused of making mistakes on purpose.

In places where bullying is commonplace, the employees won't feel like they are treated equally and often they won't even get along with each other. Employees will not enjoy the work that they do, and this will lead to a higher amount of dissatisfaction and turnover.

Some of the corporate cultural markers for bullying happen in organizations where:

- There is a high amount of pressure to make the numbers or reach the goal without worrying about the costs.
- A focus on the short-term results and not the long-term health of the employees.
- Using fear as a main motivating force.
- A high amount of cronyism.
- Inconsistent discipline procedures and appraisal processes.

Bullying in the workplace causes more problems than just high turnover. People who are bullied at work will often suffer from chronic physical illnesses. This can cause them to miss work and fall behind, which leads to further bullying. These illnesses can manifest as repeated flu or colds, but workplace bullying can also lead to more serious health concerns like heart attack, panic attacks, depression, and even PTSD.

If you are being bullied at your workplace, you might think that your only option is to quit, but there are actually many things that you can do to try and shift that negative atmosphere. As an employee in the United States, you do have certain rights.

Here are some tips to stop bullying in your workplace and keep your job:

- **Tell your story.** Find out who you need to talk to about what you are experiencing. This might be your boss, your boss' boss, or someone in Human Resources. You should have a chain of command that you can follow to someone that can help you.

- **Keep clear records.** Yes, you are going to have to report what is going on, but to do that you need to have a clear and concise story. It is vital that you write down every time you experience bullying. Keep a detailed record of the event, what was said, and who might have witnessed the abuse. By keeping a log of the bullying, you are going to have an easier time showing exactly what was inappropriate in how you were treated.

- **Don't be emotional.** Of course, you are going to have emotional reactions to what has been happening to you at the workplace, but it is important when you sit down to report it that you remain calm, cool, and collected.

- **Don't give too much information.** Only talk about what is related to the bullying behavior. Don't talk about anything that isn't connected to those actions and avoid giving your personal feelings about the person who has been bullying you. Stick to the facts.

- **Be understanding.** If you express that you understand this other employee might not realize how they are coming across, you are going to be more level-headed. Even if you don't truly believe that they don't understand their actions, it is important that you remain calm and open-minded.

THE BULLYING BASICS
A QUICK REFERENCE GUIDE

There is a lot of information to go through about bullying. It could take you a long time to fully understand what bullying is, what the implications of bullying are, and what you can do about it. Here is a handy reference of things to help you get the straight answers around bullying and what you can do about it.

WHAT BULLYING IS

- Bullying is intentional. No matter what excuses the bully may give, they always know what they are doing. Their intention is to harm the victim, either with actions or words.

- Bullying is something that happens repeatedly with a pattern; it isn't just one isolated incident. It is the repeated harassment which is what makes bullying so horrible. People who are bullied live in fear of not knowing when an attack will come.

- Bullying can be carried out by one person against another individual or it can be a group attack against one individual.

- Bullying comes in two forms, direct and indirect bullying. One is physical aggression, and the other is more manipulative emotional or mental abuse.

- Anyone at any time and any place can be bullied.

What Bullying Is Not

- Bullying is not the same thing as rough-housing or playing. It is an act of aggression against another person.

- Bullying is not something that only happens to one gender or type of person.

- Bullying is not something that only happens to other people's kids.

- Bullying is not something to ignore, brush off, or think it will just go away on its own.

What You Can Do About Bullying

- The most important thing that can be done about bullying is education. Educating kids, teachers, and parents before bullying starts has proven to be the best way to avoid it from happening altogether.

- Set good examples for your children. Don't use violence in your home. Learn to have healthy and positive means of communicating with others and be a good role model. Your kids will repeat the behavior that they see you expressing in the home.

- Report it to the school. Don't assume that the school knows what is going on. As soon as you know something is up with your child, whether they are the bully or the target, you need to let someone at the school know. The only way they will be able to make sure the bullying stops is if they know it is happening in the first place.

- Teach your kids how to handle a bullying situation. This means showing them what to do if they are bullied and what they should do if they see someone else being bullied. Most often this means teaching your kids how to stand up for themselves and instilling strong self-esteem.

Statistics About Bullying
- It is estimated by the National Education Association that nearly 160,000 children miss school every day due to intimidation or fear of attack from another student.
- According to National School Safety Center, there are somewhere around 2.1 million bullies and 2.7 million victims in the American school system.

- Over 250,000 students are attacked physically every month in secondary school.

- One out of 20 students has been reported for bringing a gun to school.

- Two-thirds of student school shootings are motivated by a desire to get back at those that bullied them.

- One out of ten high school dropouts does so because of repeated bullying.

- In a 2005 survey, students said that most of their peers had been bullied due to their physical appearance. The second top reason for bullying was due to a perceived alternative sexual orientation or gender expression.

- Half of all American teens say that they have been bullied online.

- 1 in 10 students has had an embarrassing or damaging picture of themselves posted on websites without their permission. Most often these photos have been taken with cell phone cameras.

- Only one out of ten teens that have been bullied online tell their parents about it.

- One out of four kids will experience bullying in one form or another at some point in their lives according to the American Justice Department.

- The Bureau of Justice reports that 46 percent of boys and 26 percent of girls admit to being in a physical fight due to bullying in one form or another.

- Two out of every three victims were bullied once or twice during a whole school year. One in five was bullied once a month. One in ten was bullied every single day.

- White females are the category that is most likely to be the victim of bullying.

- 10 percent of high school students have had hate terms used against them.

- 7 percent of students avoid certain places on the school campus because they are afraid of being bullied.

- Bullying is most common for middle school students.

- Students with disabilities are more likely to be bullied than children without disabilities.

In closing, bullying is a very serious problem that every parent needs to address before it gets out of control. Martial arts training, as a confidence builder for children, has shown to reduce bullying incidents drastically.

Although I do not advocate violence as a solution, I do highly recommend that a child learns how to protect themselves physically. In a last resort self-defense situation, your child must be able to protect himself or herself physically, mentally, and emotionally. Unfortunately, for many bullies, this is the only language they understand... prepare your child accordingly.

MORE BULLYING TRAGEDIES – REAL LIFE STORIES

Below are other tragic stories of victims who fell prey to vicious cyberbullying:

David Molak (2000-2016). David Molak, a sophomore at Alamo Heights High School in Texas, a fitness enthusiast, Spurs fan, and an Eagle Scout, hung himself in his family's back yard in January, 2016. His 24-year-old brother Cliff Molak, posted following the suicide: "In today's age, bullies don't push you into lockers, they don't tell their victims to meet them behind the school's dumpster after class. They cower behind user names and fake profiles from miles away constantly berating and abusing good, innocent people."

David had been the target of ongoing bullying at Alamo Heights High School. He received a series of text messages from between six and 10 bullies, with comments that put him down and insulted him. According to his brother, the bullies went after him for no reason. "He did not do anything to them besides having an attractive girlfriend. ... They crushed his spirit and took away his motivation to do anything,". Cliff also wrote the following strong words: "I saw the pain in David's eyes three nights ago as he was added to a group text only to be made fun of and kicked out two minutes later. I spoke to him right after to comfort him and he didn't even hear me. He stared off into the distance for what seemed like an hour. I could feel his pain. It was a tangible pain. He didn't even have the contact information of any of the eight members who started the group text. It is important to note David had been enduring this sort of abuse for a very long time."

*　　*　　*　　*　　*

Rachael Neblett. Rachael Neblett, a seventeen-year old high school student from Kentucky began receiving threatening emails through her MySpace account, in the summer of 2006. The anonymous emails were of a stalking terroristic nature.

Rachael's parents brought the emails to the attention of the principal of her high school. As the emails included details of her movements during class and after school, it was obvious that the bully was another student at the school.

In October Rachael received an email stating "I am not going to put you in the hospital, I am going to put you in the morgue." After receiving that email, Rachael did not want to go to school or go out with her friends.
On October 9, shortly after receiving the threatening email, Rachael took her own life. Peyton, Rachael's older sister writes:

"My little sister committed suicide October 9, 2006. Her name is Rachael Neblett. I am here to tell you a little about her. She was 17 when she died, and the most amazing girl you would ever meet. She was an out-going, loving, and caring person. You would never dream that she would do that to herself. She was not just my sister, she was my best friend ... All I have now is a big, black hole where my heart was. Because my little sister is gone, I won't be able to see her anymore--no more trips to the mall, no more smiles, hugs, late movie nights, nothing. It's gone."

*   *   *   *   *

Hope Witsell. Hope Witsell was a 13-year-old who grew up in Sundance, Florida. Her only crime was forwarding a nude photo of herself to a boy she liked. Another girl borrowed the boy's phone, found the image and forwarded it to other students. And so, the image found its way to a lot of other students in her school and in other schools. The result – taunting and bullying from her peers at Beth Shields Middle School, with insults such as "whore" and "slut".

Hope wrote in her journal. "Tons of people talk about me behind my back and I hate it because they call me a whore! And I can't be a whore I'm too inexperienced. So secretly TONS of people hate me ... " School authorities found out about the nude photo around the end of the school year and suspended Hope for the first week of eighth grade, which started in August. When she returned to school, a counselor observed cuts on Hope's legs and had her sign a "no-harm" contract, in which Hope agreed to tell an adult if she felt inclined to hurt herself. The next day, Hope hanged herself in her bedroom.

On Sept. 12, 2009, Hope wrote in her journal: "I'm done for sure now. I can feel it in my stomach. I'm going to try and strangle myself. I hope it works."

Sources: CBS, CNN and ABC News

*   *   *   *   *

These are just a few of the tragic stories that are out there. The sad part is that they could have all been prevented. It is critical that parents and teachers keep their "ears to the ground" and continue to communicate to the children and students about the damaging effects of bullying.

I hope that you found this book easy to read and resourceful. You are now armed with the knowledge to:

- Identify a bully.
- The warning signs of your child being a victim of bullying.
- Steps to take to help keep your child from becoming a bully, a victim, or a bystander.

I encourage you to use this valuable information to protect your child as he/she navigates their way through their childhood experiences. Yes, boys will be boys; however, negatively affecting one's life through consistent acts of bullying isn't the norm. Don't let society's acceptance of certain social issues convince you that it's okay – it's not okay! It's your child that we're talking about that can be negatively affected by any act of bullying – as the victim or as the bully.

As parents, teachers, and community leaders, our job is to ensure that our children are given the opportunity to grow and thrive in order to pursue their life goals and dreams without being sidetracked or emotionally scarred for life by the vicious cycle of bullying.

After all, it's their God-given right.

BULLYING

IT WON'T
END
UNLESS
YOU DO
SOMETHING
ABOUT IT

About the Author

Samuel Scott (known as Master Scott to his students and peers) is the founder of Full Circle Martial Arts Academy (Capitol Heights, MD). He has studied martial arts for over 42 years in which he began his school in the basement of his home in 1992. For the last 25 years, Master Scott has dedicated his life to developing our future leaders through the teachings of martial excellence.

As a 15-year veteran of the Prince George's Dept. of Corrections (Upper Marlboro, MD), he has seen first-hand, both the results of kids being a bully and kids being the victims of bullying. What he learned as a Correction Officer is that, often, those that grew up as bullies found themselves heavily involved in drugs, excessive alcohol use, domestic abuse, and other violent crimes. Unfortunately, this was also the same situation for many victims of bullying. (However, he also notes that many teens were locked-up for merely following the wrong crowd.)

Per Master Scott, it appeared that many of the victims, due to their childhood experience with bullying, had a need or desire to be a part of the tough crowd. With this insight, Master Scott started an unrelenting mission to reach out to our future leaders and arm them with a deep love for self, strong character skills, and rock-solid confidence. Although Master Scott has accomplished much in the martial arts world like:

- Black Belt Hall of Fame Inductee.
- Author of seven books.
- Gold Medal winner in the 1992 International Police Olympics.

- Top-rank fighter with over 300 fights.
- Inductee in the International Who's Who in the Martial Arts (and featured in the book with martial arts icons such as actors Michael J. White, actress Cynthia Rothrock, and actor Don ("the Dragon") Wilson, and hundreds more).
- Awarded a 3-year contract to train the Abu Dhabi Police.
- As of 2017, created over 140 Black Belts (in which most were kids when they started).

He feels that his greatest accomplishment has been his ability to transform thousands of people's lives both here and abroad. Master Scott has dedicated his entire life to creating future leaders out of our young people. So, this book is just another way for him to reach the parents and teachers of our future leaders to help bring an end to this vicious cycle of behavior, together.

Master Scott's commitment to empowering the community with skills to thrive and to protect and preserve human kindness is real. Read and share this book, *The Bully Problem: Don't Leave Your Child's Future in The Hands of A Bully*, and join him in his fight to put an end to bullying!

RESOURCES

(To help you monitor your child's activity while on the phone and computer.)

(Resource: www.parents.com)

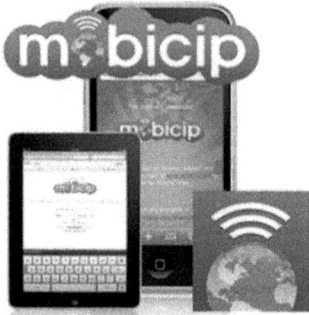

Mobicip (Mobile App)

In 2010, Mobicip was awarded the 2010 Parents' Choice Silver Honors Award for top mobile app filtering. There are three restriction levels: for kids. It includes a wide array of parental controls, including category blocking, time limits, Internet activity reports, blocked phrases, and YouTube. The elementary school level blocks social networking, gaming, shopping, entertainment, clothing, and news content. The middle school level blocks online shopping, gambling, dating, liquor, and chat sites. The high school level blocks adult, sexual, weapons, violence, proxy, virus, and hacking sites.

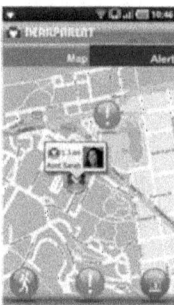

NearParent (Mobile App)

NearParent allows families to build a trusted network of adults who can assist children when they are in need. The app has three views -- "kid's," "alert," and "helper's." In the "kid's view," a child who requires assistance clicks either a "small alert" or "urgent alert" button on the app, which then notifies adults in his network that help is needed. The "alert view" reveals the adult helper who will provide assistance and the "helper's view" reveals the child's and the helper's locations to determine how far they are from each other. **(Free; iPhone, iPad)**

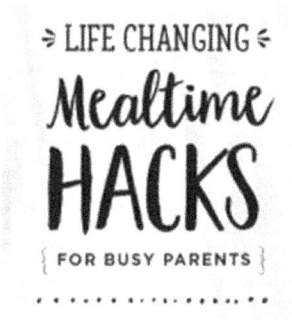

Genius Mealtime Hacks for Busy Parents

These meal prep tips will improve your productivity in a HUGE way. Busy parents: This guide is for you!

PROVIDED BY QUAKER® OVERNIGHT OATS

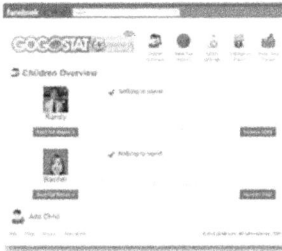

Courtesy of GoGoStat's Parental Guidance

GoGoStat's Parental Guidance (Mobile App)

This app lets you see posts from your kids containing drug references and vulgarities, know when they post photos and profile details that should not be public, and check when they add new friends that are out of a predetermined age or geographic range. Parents can also print social media Emergency Reports, developed with the help of law enforcement. **(Free; iPhone, iPad)**

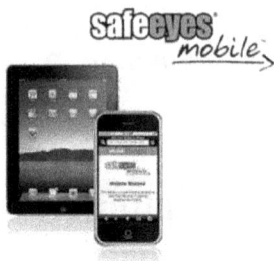

Safe Eyes Mobile (Mobile App)

Control your child's Internet usage while she's on the iPhone by blocking questionable sites. This app has YouTube filtering and media player blocking. You can also customize it by choosing from 35 different categories (e.g., nudity, profanity, etc.) to block or allow content.

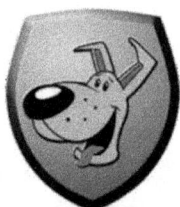

My Mobile Watchdog (Mobile and Web App)

Get alerts on your mobile phone and computer that include updates about questionable texts, photos, videos, and unauthorized phone numbers. Parents can work with their child to create a master contact list for his mobile phone, but only parents can add or make changes. **(fee-based)**

CyberSynchs' Parental Mode (Mobile Cloud)

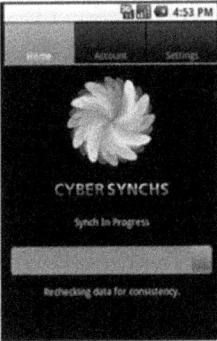

CyberSynchs is an innovative service that allows mobile users to back up, share, and synchronize data between the phone and the computer. Its Parental Mode setting allows parents to receive reports that have blurbs of content with flagged words that indicate bullying, sexual behavior, and violence. Parents can also prevent access to certain synchronized data and view the child's last GPS location. **(fee-based)**

Net Nanny (Mobile App and Software)

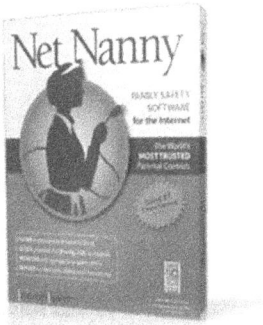

Notification monitors send alerts when alarming keywords are used. The best part: You program those words in advance. There is time control, to limit when and for how long kids can access the internet, plus a setup assistant that allows parents to determine which online sites are appropriate for the child's age. A mobile app version is also available for Android phones only. **(fee-based)**

Trend Micro's Online Guardian for Families (Software)

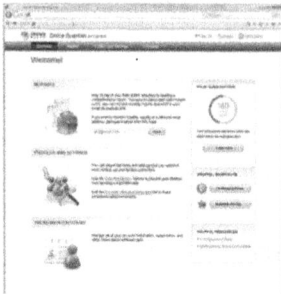

A mom who witnessed her daughter being cyberbullied started Online Guardian, which contains extensive controls (on an easy centralized dashboard) for tracking social networking sites (Twitter, Facebook, Flickr, YouTube, and MySpace), instant messaging management, and malware protection. **(fee-based)**

SafetyWeb (Software)

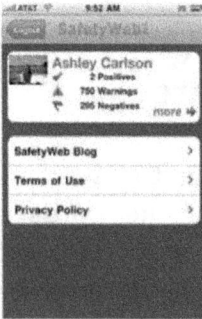

Track your child's activity on social networking sites, and monitor text and instant messages. Parents can receive a free sample report after typing a child's email address on the product's site to see what comes up in an Internet search. The site offers a money-back guarantee, and subscribers have free access to the mobile version. **(fee-based)**

YouDiligence (Software)

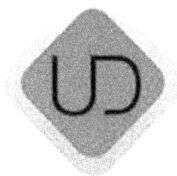

YOUDiligence™

Responsible social networking.

If your child has a social networking account, monitor his page and track keywords related to bullying, racial slurs, alcohol, cursing, and more. YouDiligence provides a list of 500 dangerous words and phrases that parents can edit, based on their values. Reports of anything problematic are then viewed via email alerts and an online dashboard. **(fee-based)**

SocialShield (Software)

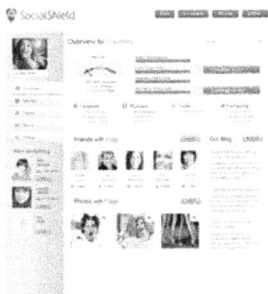

Founded by two men who heard their friend's daughter received unwanted attention from a male adult on Facebook, SocialShield monitors social networking sites (Facebook, MySpace, Twitter) to protect a child's online reputation. By using cloud-based software, it can be accessed anywhere via computer and phone. Reports provide a safety score on a scale of 1 to 10 (10 being the safest) that is determined by reputation-harming watchwords in posts and discussions, photos, videos, and friends. **(fee-based)**

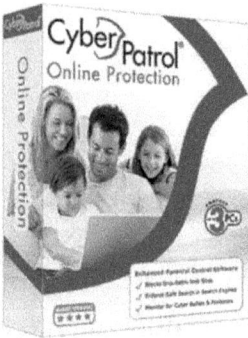

Cyber Patrol Online Protection (Software)

Awarded the Parent Tested Parent Approved (PTPA) seal of approval, Cyber Patrol has several computer software programs that protect kids' internet safety. The Online Protection software sends "Bully Alerts" that scan for language that indicates cyberbullying. Parents can set up time limits for when children can go online, block questionable sites and programs, and receive daily and weekly summaries of Internet activities. **(fee-based)**

www.ingramcontent.com/pod-product-compliance
Lightning Source LLC
Chambersburg PA
CBHW072134020426
42334CB00018B/1803